FUNK & WAGNALLS
NEW ILLUSTRATED ENCYCLOPEDIA OF
FAMILY HEALTH

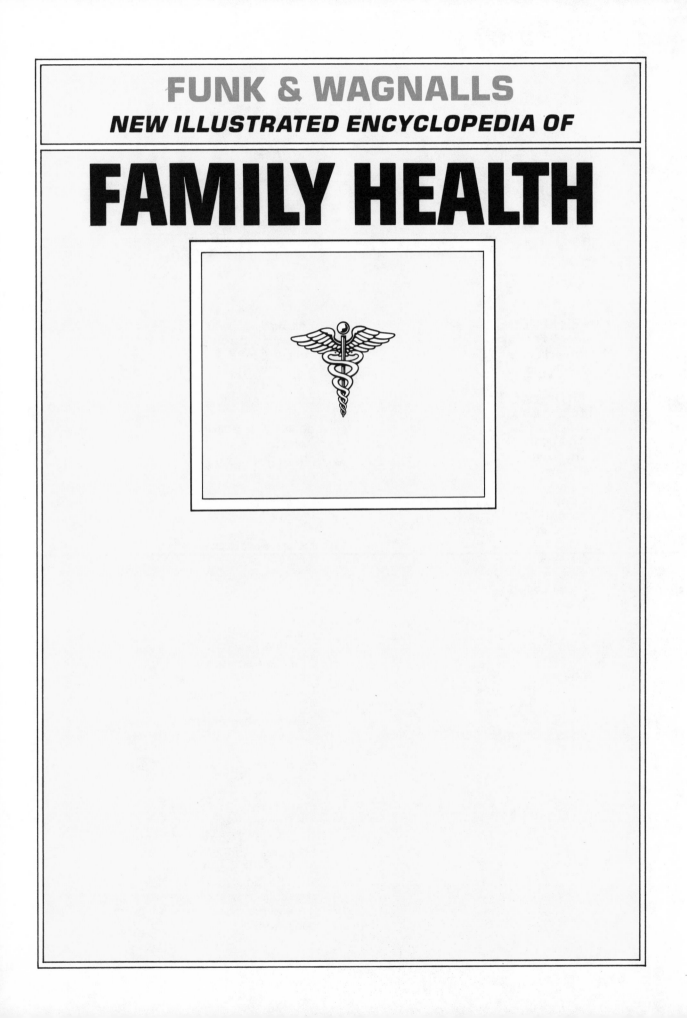

REFERENCE EDITION

Project Editor
Sarah Bourne

Art Director
Keith Vollans

Art Editors
Kay Carroll
B Syme

Copy Editors
Penny Smith
Caroline Macy
Fiona Wilson
Jill Wiley

Index Editor
Theresa Donaghey

Managing Editor
Alan Ross

Editorial Director
Maggi McCormick

Production
Carol Milligan

Editors
Edward Horton
Felicity Smart

Deputy Editor
Elizabeth Longley

Senior Sub-editors
Anna Bradley
Sheila Brull
Arlene Sobel

Art Editor
Maggie Howells

Picture Researchers
Julia Calloway
Elizabeth Strachan
Vickie Walters

Designers
Pamela Alvares
Shirin Patel
Chris Rathbone
Jervis Tuttle
Ginger Wetherley

Artwork Researcher
Sally Walters

Production Executive
Robert Paulley

Chief Editorial Consultant
Dr. Trevor Weston,
Founder and Chairman of Health
Education Audio-Visual and Consultant
Medical Editor of the British Medical
Association's *Family Doctor*
Publications Unit. He has been both a
general practitioner and a hospital
consultant.

FUNK & WAGNALLS
NEW ILLUSTRATED ENCYCLOPEDIA OF
FAMILY HEALTH

VOLUME
1

MARSHALL CAVENDISH · LONDON · SYDNEY · NEW YORK
Distributed by Funk & Wagnalls, Inc., Ramsey, NJ

Reference Edition Published 1988
© Marshall Cavendish Limited
MCMLXXXI, MCMLXXXII, MCMLXXXIII,
MCMLXXXVI, MCMLXXXVIII

ISBN 0-86307-869-9 (Set)
ISBN 0-86307-870-2 (Vol 1)

Distributed by Funk & Wagnalls, Inc.,
Ramsey, NJ.

FUNK & WAGNALLS and F & W are
registered trademarks of Funk &
Wagnalls, Inc.

Distributed to schools and libraries by
Marshall Cavendish Corporation.

**Library of Congress Cataloging
in Publication Data**

Funk & Wagnalls new illustrated
    encyclopedia of family health.

    Rev. ed. of: The Marshall Cavendish
illustrated encyclopedia of family health.
1984.
    Includes index.
    1. Medicine, Popular—Dictionaries. I.
Funk & Wagnalls. II. Marshall
Cavendish illustrated encyclopedia of
family health. III. Title: Funk and
Wagnalls new illustrated encyclopedia
of family health.
RC81.F95 1988   610'.3'21   87-23663
ISBN 0-86307-869-9 (set)

Printed in the United States of America.

Published by Marshall Cavendish House
58 Old Compton Street
London WIV 5PA

INTRODUCTION

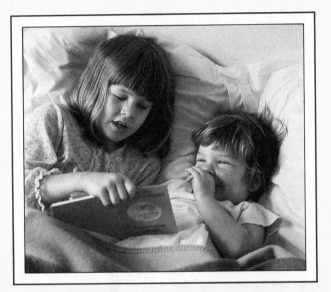

Our health is our most precious asset — and the health of our families is quite properly a major concern. The *Funk & Wagnalls New Illustrated Encyclopedia of Family Health* has been specially prepared to fill a unique role in this most crucial area. It is a complete and authoritative guide to your family's health, prepared by a team of experts but written in language that is clear, untechnical and straight to the point.

In every volume you will find the answers to the sort of questions you are most likely to ask, so it's really like having your own family doctor permanently on call. Not, of course, that the *Funk & Wagnalls New Illustrated Encyclopedia of Family Health* is in any sense a substitute for the enormous range of services provided by the medical profession. But doctors tell us that knowledge is the key to preventing ill health — knowledge of how our body works, knowledge of what we should and should not do to keep it in the best possible working order, and, perhaps most important of all, the knowledge that enables us to recognise any illness or disorder in its earliest stages, when medical treatment stands the greatest chance of success.

In more than 900 individual articles, arranged alphabetically for easy reference, our experts give you the inside information — dispelling myths and fallacies and replacing them with hard facts, the facts you need at your fingertips to cope with everyday health care. Each article features a special section giving the 'Doctor's' straightforward answers to the most relevant questions. Each article is fully illustrated in colour with photographs, informative diagrams and charts, to help in getting the subject across quickly, accurately, and above all, in a manner that is easily understood. A fully cross-referenced index closes Volume 23.

Volume 24 contains a quick-reference First Aid Handbook, an extensive glossary of medical terms, a complete listing of articles by volume and a classified listing of articles to help you get the most from this valuable work.

PREFACE

For most doctors, establishing a strong relationship with their patients is one of the greatest rewards of practising medicine. Regrettably most of us are unable to spend as much time as we would like with each patient — explaining exactly what is happening to their bodies or providing a detailed account of the precise effect a given treatment is going to have.

This is why I welcome the publication of the *Funk & Wagnalls New Illustrated Encyclopedia of Family Health,* a reliable guide you can turn to for advice and reassurance any time you have a question about your health. It is especially helpful to consult before you visit your doctor's office, so that you can use the time wisely by asking the most informed questions, and then afterwards in case you have any questions you forgot to ask, would like more information, want to clear up any point you didn't understand, or need a reminder of what your doctor told you.

However, this encyclopedia is not intended to be a 'do-it-yourself' medical kit, and it most certainly cannot replace your own doctor. While every care has been taken to ensure that the information presented here is in accord with current medical knowledge, personal circumstances vary so enormously that it is not possible to be sure that all the advice given is right for every individual. Consequently, if you have any particular worry about your health, it is important to consult your doctor about it, as well as making use of the guidance *Funk & Wagnalls New Illustrated Encyclopedia of Family Health* can give you.

Trevor Weston, MD, MRCGP
Chief Editorial Consultant

CONTENTS

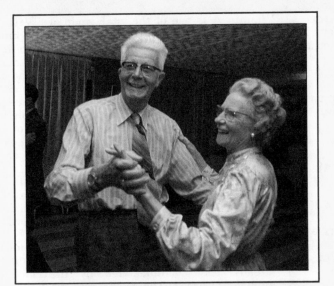

A-vitamin

Q What are vitamins? Are they really important?

A Vitamins are organic substances present in minute amounts in food. Put simply, they help make our bodies work. Because they cannot be made by the body, vitamins must be obtained from the diet. We require only very small amounts of them, but they are absolutely essential to normal metabolism, and a serious deficiency will inevitably lead to disease.

Q Should I take vitamin supplements to make sure I don't develop a vitamin deficiency?

A Children, the elderly, pregnant women and nursing mothers, as well as people recovering from an illness, may need a supplement of certain vitamins. A healthy adult, though, will usually obtain enough through a well-balanced diet.

Q I know a daily dose of halibut liver oil is good for children. Is a double dose twice as good?

A Halibut liver oil is a valuable source of vitamin A, but it is dangerous to exceed the recommended dose. Because vitamin A is stored in the body, excessive amounts can be toxic.

Q I've heard that vitamin A helps prevent colds. Is there any truth to this?

A Vitamin A aids the body in producing mucus-secreting cells, and this is one of the ways the body protects itself from germs. It works by removing them from the body—by the nose in the case of a cold. So a lack of vitamin A could make you more likely to catch colds.

Q Will eating carrots help me see in the dark, or is this just an old wives' tale?

A There is some truth in this old wives' tale. The carotene contained in carrots provides vitamin A, which helps your eyes to adjust to dim light quickly.

We have all heard of vitamins and know they are essential for good health. But what are they, what do they do and, among them, just how important is vitamin A?

Vitamin A is one of the vital group of vitamins that the body needs to function properly. It enables us to see in a dim light, keeps our skin healthy, ensures normal growth and renews the body tissue. With only a few exceptions, we obtain all the vitamins we need from our food, and the minute amounts the body requires mostly exist in their natural state in food. But vitamin A is largely manufactured by the body from a food substance called carotene.

Sources of vitamin A
The vitamin A in our food comes in two different forms from two different sources. The pure form, called retinol, is found in foods such as fish-liver oils, liver, kidney, cheese, eggs and butter, having already been manufactured by the animal concerned. The second form we make ourselves from carotene, which is found in such vegetables as carrots, spinach, cabbage, and tomatoes.

In fact, when a vegetable is orange, yellow or dark green in colour, what you are seeing is its carotene content, and the darker the green of the vegetable, the greater the carotene content. Spinach and watercress therefore contain more in each pound than cabbage, and dark green cabbage provides more than lighter types of vegetable.

Carotene is converted into retinol in the liver and in the small intestine, and then some of the vitamin A—whether it be converted carotene or retinol itself—is absorbed into the blood stream and circulated round the body to be used in its everyday functions, while the rest is stored in the liver.

Although vitamin A is not present in many foods, those which contain it are fortunately readily available. A fifth of our average intake comes from vegetables, mainly carrots. Turnips and potatoes are no substitute, however, since they contain no carotene. Milk and butter are other common sources; margarine, to which vitamin A is added artificially, contains almost as much as butter and is therefore just as good.

Vitamin A-rich foods tend not to lose their vitamin content easily, though prolonged exposure to light and air can reduce the amount. Cooking at normal temperatures has no serious effect, but frying at a relatively high temperature in butter or margarine will result in some loss of vitamin content.

Vitamin A deficiency
Itching, burning and reddened eyelids are among the problems caused by lack of vitamin A, and a drastic deficiency can lead to blindness. The children of the poorer nations are often vulnerable and a cause is early weaning on to an unsuitable food like skimmed milk, which can contain little or no vitamin A. However prepared baby foods almost always have essential vitamins added to them.

In our more affluent society our diet is better balanced, and most of us get as much vitamin A as we need, about two thirds of it coming from retinol and one third from carotene.

But even so, a deficiency of vitamin A can cause night blindness. Doctors have long recognized night blindness as a medical condition. Normally, it takes about seven to ten minutes for your eyes to become used to a dim light—so if you are dazzled for some time after seeing another car's headlights at night, or if you find it difficult to distinguish objects in the semi-dark, see your doctor to find out if you have vitamin A deficiency. Taking halibut liver oil capsules is the quickest cure, as it is one of the best sources of vitamin A.

If you are on a high protein diet you could risk a deficiency simply because the body uses up the vitamin much faster when converting protein into body tissue and energy. But there are other times when the body uses up its store of vitamin A too quickly, such as when there is a high fever.

Taking certain drugs also causes a loss. Your doctor will advise you as to how much vitamin A is needed should any of these situations arise.

Excessive vitamin A
The forty or so vitamins can be divided into two types—those that can be stored by the body and those that cannot. As vitamin A is stored in the liver, daily intake is not essential though regular supplies are needed. There is some danger however in taking too much vitamin A. This is very unlikely to result from intake through food but can occur if large amounts are taken in concentrated forms such as halibut liver oil capsules. Symptoms may include insomnia, weight loss, dryness of the lips, and aching limbs. But, in general, taking slightly more than is needed is unlikely to harm you or your child.

Vitamin A—Are you getting enough?

The daily requirement for different age groups and the vitamin A content in the foods listed are given in micrograms (1,000 micrograms = one milligram, or one thousandth of a gram).

There is no need to worry if you are unable to take the correct amount every day as long as the amount you take over a week gives the correct daily average.

Age group		Daily requirement
Babies under 12 months		450
Children	1-6	300
	7-8	400
	9-11	575
Adolescents		750
Adult men and women		750
Expectant mothers		
first 4 months		750
until the birth		900
during breastfeeding		1,200

Food	Vitamin A content
Apricots, dried, 57 g (2 oz)	340
Butter, 28 g (1 oz)	282
Cabbage, 114 g (4 oz)	56
Carrots, 114 g (4 oz)	2267
Cheese, 57 g (2 oz)	238
Cod liver oil capsule, 1	180
Cream, heavy, 2 tablespoons (30 ml)	130
Egg, 1	80
Halibut liver oil capsule, 1	1200

Food	Vitamin A content
Kidney, 114 g (4 oz)	340
Fish, oily, 114 g (4 oz)	52
Liver, ox, 114 g (4 oz)	6800
Margarine, 28 g (1 oz)	255
Milk, whole, .2 L (7 fl oz)	80
Peas, frozen, 114 g (4 oz)	56
Prunes, dried, 57 g (2 oz)	90
Spinach, 114 g (4 oz)	1136
Tomato, 42 g (1½ oz)	49
Watercress, 28 g (1 oz)	142

Di Lewis

Abdomen

Q I went for a job interview the other day and my tummy rumbled all the time. I was so embarrassed. As I didn't get the job, how can I avoid the problem next time?

A Tummy rumblings go on all the time as the intestine churns and digests food, but cannot usually be heard except through a stethoscope. Louder rumblings tend to occur when the intestine is empty or contains too much air. You were probably a little bit nervous at the prospect of your interview, and when people are nervous they often swallow air without realizing it. So next time, have a good meal before you set off, try to relax and suck a peppermint or two to help prevent you from air swallowing.

Q My child often complains of a tummy ache on Monday mornings. It seems odd that it's only then. Is she just shamming?

A Quite probably she does have a real pain in her abdomen caused not by some sort of infection but by nerves. The pain, though real, is probably caused by a mental rather than a physical problem. Try to find out why Mondays are so much to be dreaded. Perhaps she is being bullied or is afraid of one of her teachers. Once you get to the root of the problems and iron out her anxieties, the trouble should disappear very quickly.

Q My baby seems to have a huge abdomen, just like one of those starving children I've seen on television. Is this normal?

A Quite normal. A baby's abdomen looks swollen because his liver is very large—it has to be to do many of the important jobs essential to growth, for example making blood—and the abdominal muscles are not yet very strong. By the time he is about five he should have lost this 'pot bellied' look. Starving children have swollen abdomens whatever their age. This is a part of a disease called kwashiorkor caused by a diet containing little or no protein. Such children do not have sturdy limbs like your baby but arms and legs so wasted that they look like matchsticks.

The abdomen is the factory area of the body, containing most of the digestive system, the urinary system and, in women, the reproductive organs. With all these activities going on inside, it is not surprising that pains in the abdomen can have a huge variety of causes.

The abdomen is the biggest cavity in the body, extending from underneath the diaphragm, the sheet of muscle that forms the lower boundary of the chest, down to the groin. Bound at the back of the body by the spine, and round its upper sides by the ribs, the front of the abdomen is covered by a thick sheet of muscle which can be felt just by 'pulling it in'. And it is easy to realize just how elastic this muscle is by picturing how much it can stretch to accommodate a baby during pregnancy.

Inside the abdomen
There are a great number of organs in the abdomen, often called the viscera. Nearly all the alimentary canal lies inside the abdomen, starting with the stomach sited just under the diaphragm and ending with the rectum, which empties out via the anus. The alimentary canal is the body's food processing system—it breaks down food into substances that can be absorbed into the blood to be carried to all parts of the body, and ejects indigestible wastes. Backing up the alimentary canal

Female abdomen with alimentary canal removed

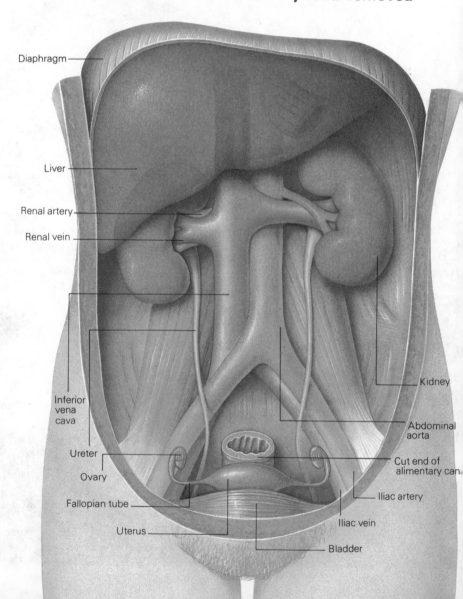

Diaphragm

Liver

Renal artery

Renal vein

Inferior vena cava

Ureter

Ovary

Fallopian tube

Uterus

Kidney

Abdominal aorta

Cut end of alimentary canal

Iliac artery

Iliac vein

Bladder

Mike Courteney

4

are important abdominal glands such as the liver and pancreas, plus the spleen, which is part of the defence system against disease. A huge network of blood vessels serves all the abdominal organs and nerves.

Behind the alimentary canal lie the kidneys, each joined by a tube called a ureter to the bladder, which is in the lower part of the abdomen and in which urine is stored before it is released. Closely connected to the urinary system is the reproductive system. In women, nearly all the sex organs are inside the abdomen, but in men part of the sex organs descend to a position outside the body before birth.

It might seem impossible for so many vital organs to be squeezed into such a comparatively small space, but through the centuries of evolution the 10 m (33 ft) or so of gut have become coiled and twisted to fit inside the abdomen. To keep everything in place, the abdomen is lined with a kind of tissue sac called the peritoneum and the organs are attached to it by sheets or strings of tissue known as mesenteries.

When something goes wrong
With so much going on inside the

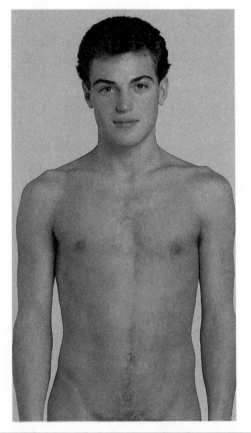

abdomen, it is perhaps just as well that, apart from the odd rumble of the intestines, it is impossible to feel each organ at work. But because we cannot feel them working, we cannot actually detect when anything goes wrong, except 'by proxy' in some other part of the body. Thus the pain of a stomach ulcer, for example, is real enough but it is not in the stomach itself that the pain is felt but in nerve signals reaching the upper part of the abdomen.

Pains in the abdomen vary in position, type and intensity according to the cause of the trouble within and are in themselves good clues for the doctor's diagnosis. The pains are usually accompanied by other symptoms—nausea, vomiting and/or diarrhoea, as for instance in the case of food poisoning. And diseases of the abdominal organs can also be detected by pains in other parts of the body such as the back and shoulders.

Sex-linked symptoms
Many women become concerned about an uncomfortable, low abdominal pain which they get midway between periods. This is in fact perfectly normal, and it isn't worth bothering the doctor with unless the pain persists for more than 24 hours or is accompanied by bleeding.

Common causes of abdominal pain

Position	Type of pain/symptoms	Possible causes	What to do
Top centre, behind breastbone	Severe discomfort, or burning sensation. Nausea and headache. Heavy feeling in abdomen which may be distended. Wind or heartburn.	Inflammation of stomach due to infection, excess of rich or spicy food, alcohol or nicotine. Peptic ulcer or chronic gastritis	Take antacids, plenty of fluids, eat a bland diet. Cut down on drinking and smoking, try to avoid stress. See your doctor if pain persists
Top centre, moving through to back	Colicky (griping), persistent or intermittent, may be relieved by food. Upper part of abdomen may feel full and be distended	Peptic ulcer or inflammation of the pancreas	Take antacids for temporary relief, plus small milky meals, but see your doctor this week
Top centre, behind ribs, moving to right	Constant, may be made worse by fatty foods. Heartburn, abdomen feels oppressively full. Possibly jaundiced	Inflamed gall bladder, inflammation of liver (hepatitis)	See your doctor today
Top centre, shooting to right shoulder	Agonizing, with sweating, nausea and vomiting	Trapped gall stones (biliary colic)	See your doctor urgently, take painkillers for temporary relief
Centre, around or above navel	Persistent, may be burning, cramping or griping, often accompanied by vomiting and/or diarrhoea. Abdomen distended	Food poisoning, gastro-enteritis or other infection of the intestine	Take plenty of fluid and kaopectate or peptobismal mixture. No food for 24 hours. See doctor if symptoms persist.
Centre or in either loin, may shoot down to groin; burning on urination	Colicky or persistent, may be worse on movement and accompanied by vomiting	Kidney infection or stone (renal colic)	See your doctor today, or at once if pain is very severe
Centre, round navel, moving to lower right	Persistent, may be accompanied by flatulence, nausea and vomiting. Constipation	Appendicitis	See your doctor today, or at once if pain is very severe. Do not take laxatives or antacids

The pain is actually caused by an increase in tension in the ovary as the egg is released halfway between each menstrual period. Many women do not have this pain at all but wish that they did—for it is quite an accurate indication of when the egg is being released and therefore when a woman is most likely to get pregnant.

Also connected with reproduction, but rather more unusual, is the set of symptoms of a sympathetic pregnancy. Occasionally it is possible for a man whose wife is pregnant to suffer some of the same symptoms as a pregnant woman. The condition is caused by extreme overanxiety, and the man suffers abdominal swelling and also sometimes morning sickness and food cravings. After the birth the abdomen invariably returns to normal.

When to seek help

Abdominal pains are something that everyone has experienced, but it is important to remember that although they often have a trivial cause, such as overeating, constipation or a mild 'tummy bug', they can be a signal that something is seriously wrong. Abdominal pain should always be taken seriously and should not just be masked with pain killers, which can actually cover up important symptoms that require a

Intestinal organs

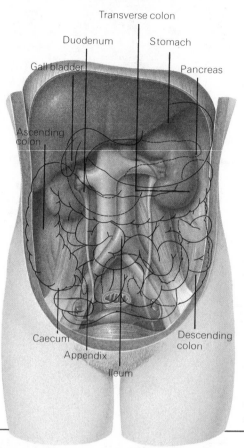

Transverse colon

Duodenum

Stomach

Gall bladder

Pancreas

Ascending colon

Caecum

Descending colon

Appendix

Ileum

doctor's immediate attention and care.

In obvious, everyday complaints, wai 48 hours before seeking medical help, bu in severe, sudden abdominal pain neve just 'grin and bear it' or take pain-killer or laxatives. If an intense pain lasts mor than a few hours, and particularly if it i accompanied by a swollen abdomen tha feels tender to the touch and by blood o tarry substances in the stool *see a docto at once*. This is most important — don feel you are wasting his time. It could be the sign of serious illness.

Treating children's pains

All the same rules apply if children have pains in the abdomen, but if in doubt always consult your doctor. In childrer abdominal pain may also result from problems uncommon in adult life. Good examples are tonsillitis, middle ear in fections and lead poisoning from chewing lead-containing paint.

Anxiety is another common cause o tummy ache in both children and adults—and results from the natura tendency of the body to intensify the squeezing action of the intestine in times of stress. If possible it is best not to eat at times like these because food is particu larly hard to digest when the abdomen is tight. But hot drinks may bring some comfort and relief.

Position	Type of pain/symptoms	Possible causes	What to do
Centre, above, around or just below navel, right or left	Griping. Abdomen may be distended. Hard stools may alternate with diarrhoea	Constipation, irritable colon, or diverticulitis	Increase bran and roughage content of diet. See your doctor if symptoms persist
Centre, around and below navel	Cramping with frequent vomiting and constipation. Abdomen distended	Intestinal obstruction	See your doctor urgently
Centre, below navel	Griping, intermittent. Abdomen may be distended	Inflammation of the colon, miscarriage or passing of a blood clot from the vagina	See your doctor today
Centre, below navel	Persistent, occurring during or just before menstruation. Abdomen may be distended	Premenstrual tension, period pain	Take pain killers but see your doctor if symptoms persist or become severe
Below navel, right or left	Persistent dull ache, worse during periods, lower abdomen may be distended	Congestion in area of the uterus, inflammation of pelvic or sex organs, venereal disease	See your doctor this week
Below navel, right or left	Colicky, intermittent, accompanying scanty or missed periods	Ectopic pregnancy (fetus lodged in the Fallopian tubes)	See your doctor today
Very low, centre, may move down into groin	Constant, may be worse as bladder fills. Burning sensation during urination, urine may be thick or contain blood	Cystitis or urinary infection	See your doctor today. Take plenty of fluids
All over abdomen	Agonizing, rapid onset, very tender all over abdomen. Generally very ill, possibly collapsed	Peritonitis from perforated peptic ulcer or burst appendix	Call a doctor or get to hospital urgently

Q How would I be able to tell whether my daughter was suffering from appendicitis, or from some other internal problem that was less serious?

A At first, the pain of an appendicitis is very difficult to distinguish from any other type of stomach ache. The pain will come and go, similar to colic, and generally it is first felt around the area of the navel. Your daughter would be uninterested in food, would probably feel sick and be constipated. A mild pain killer can be given at this stage and perhaps some warm milk. After about six to 12 hours, if it is appendicitis, the pain will increase and is usually concentrated down the lower right hand side of the abdomen. It would be very painful by this time. A rise in temperature, vomiting and bad breath, combined with extreme pain, are definite indications of suspected appendicitis and the doctor should be called.

Q The first meal I ate after a bout of diarrhoea and sickness gave me violent pains in my stomach. Why was this?

A It sounds as if you ate too heavy a meal too soon after your sickness. You must remember that when you have had something like gastro-enteritis, the lining of your stomach becomes very tender. You should have allowed your stomach to rest. After an attack of such symptoms, including food poisoning, you should mainly drink fluids and eat only light, bland foods for a few days.

Q Recently, I have been suffering from very bad pains in my upper abdomen just after eating my breakfast and I have quite a lot of acid-indigestion throughout the day. What could be causing this?

A Any persistent symptoms such as yours should be checked by a doctor. However, if you are a heavy smoker and drinker you could be aggravating inflammation of your stomach. Other conditions which can cause severe abdominal pain such as you describe can include a stomach ulcer, kidney stones or gallstones.

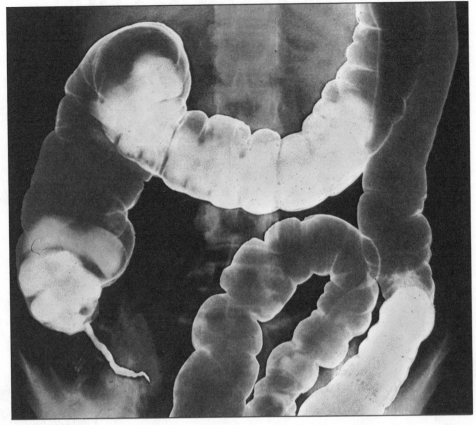

Science Photo Library

False-colour x-ray of the abdomen showing the large intestine (colon). Barium sulphate has been injected into the rectum.

Examining the abdomen

A doctor can diagnose many disorders of the abdomen simply by 'palpating' (examining by touch) the surface of the skin over the affected area. For example, an enlarged liver can clearly be felt on the outside of the abdomen. Similarly, many problems of the female reproductive system can be diagnosed manually by conventional internal examination.

However, in many cases, for a complete diagnosis, the doctor uses a number of tests, involving X-rays, scans and the use of flexible fibroptic tubes.

X-rays

Since X-rays normally pass through internal organs, a contrast medium must be used to produce a clear image. The contrast can be given intravenously (by injection into a vein), by mouth or via the anus in an enema.

Cholangiography, in which the contrast is either injected into a vein or directly into the liver, is used to examine the gall bladder, bile ducts and liver. The duodenum can be X-rayed by duodenography, when the contrast is given through a catheter passed via the mouth into the duodenum. And, in the upper and lower GI series, barium is given either by mouth (barium milkshake or swallow) or as an enema to X-ray the oesophagus, stomach and intestines.

Scans

Radioisotope scanning, also called nuclear scanning, involves the use of a small amount of radioactive material which is injected into a vein. This sounds alarming, but the amount of radiation is very low and there is very little risk of isotope overdose. Radiation enables the concentration of various hormones and minerals in the internal organs to be scanned to indicate possible malfunctions. Both the liver and pancreas can be examined in this way.

Fibroptic examination

By passing a flexible fibroptic tube into the body, a doctor can literally see the internal organs. In colonoscopy, the tube is passed through the rectum to check for polyps or ulcers in the bowels. Similarly, gastroscopy allows the doctor to make a visual examination of the stomach and upper part of the small intestine for ulcers, tumours and possible causes of internal bleeding. In this case, the tube is passed through the mouth and esophagus. And in woman, a laparascope may be inserted through the wall of the abdomen so the doctor can look directly at the womb, fallopian tubes and ovaries.

Abrasions and cuts

Q Is it better to cover wounds or let them heal in the open air?

A As a general rule, all wet, weepy wounds need covering. Most fresh wounds are best protected if you are working in dirty conditions, but dry wounds should be left uncovered in clean conditions.

Q Do old people heal as quickly as the young?

A Generally, older bodies heal just as quickly as young ones, but there are a few exceptions. Sometimes arterial disease diminishes the blood flow and makes healing a slow process. Infection is more likely and ulcers may develop, especially on the shins and ankles, where circulation is often bad. Cuts on an elderly person's leg need prompt, daily attention if ulcers are to be avoided.

Q If a limb is bleeding severely, should I try to make a tourniquet?

A Tourniquets—strips of cloth or other material wrapped tightly around a limb—stop bleeding by cutting off the blood supply. They were once widely used but are now thought to be dangerous because a low blood and oxygen level in any limb can cause permanent damage and make infection more likely. Tourniquets should only be used by a qualified person.

Q Do I need a tetanus injection every time I get cut?

A Like most people you will probably have been immunized against tetanus as a child. Immunization involves having a series of three injections within a year. To maintain protection you should have a booster every ten years. If you have not had one in the last ten years (five years if the wound is very serious) you will need to have a small booster injection if you are cut. An injection is particularly important if you were cut while gardening or in the countryside, as the bacteria which cause tetanus live in soil and animal manure. If you are uncertain whether you have been immunized seek medical advice. Tetanus germs cause lockjaw, a very serious condition that is often fatal.

The skin protects vulnerable internal organs from injury, but as the body's front line of defence it often gets damaged itself. Fast, effective first aid can help speed the healing process and prevent infection.

Scratches, abrasions, cuts, lacerations and punctures are all abnormal breaks through the skin and are generally referred to as wounds. The body itself has very efficient mechanisms for staunching bleeding, healing wounds and fighting infection, but it often needs help. Whenever the skin is broken blood vessels may be torn and germs can enter the body, so all wounds need to be cleaned and many need to be dressed.

How the body copes

Blood contains special proteins that form a protective mesh of strands and cells when tissue is damaged. Called a blood clot, it seals off the broken blood vessels and stops bleeding. At the same time the muscles in the walls of the damaged blood vessels contract to slow down the flow of blood. If bleeding is severe the blood pressure is lowered throughout the body.

Also, as soon as skin is broken, special white blood cells called phagocytes gather at the site of injury. They remove any microscopic particles like bacteria and so are the body's first line of defence against infection. As expected, the larger the damaged area the more likely it will be contaminated with bacteria and the greater the chance of infection.

When bleeding has stopped and the wound is clear of infection, a fibrous scab begins to form. The scab shrinks over the next few days and forms an extremely strong bond between the cut surfaces.

Stopping the bleeding is usually the first concern with any wound. If simply applying pressure with a clean cloth to an arm or leg wound is not effective, try to locate a pressure point— inside the upper arm or leg—and press firmly.

Di Lewis

8

First aid for minor injuries

How to stop bleeding

Sometimes it is better to allow a wound to bleed for a while because the flow of blood can help to wash dirt and bacteria away. This is particularly important with a puncture wound, as these are very difficult to clean properly. However if bleeding is profuse, it should be stopped.

Unless you suspect a broken limb, in which case the limb should not be moved, raise the limb so that the blood pressure is reduced slightly.

Then, using a clean bandage, apply firm pressure to the wound. The pressure needs to be constant for at least five minutes to be effective. If blood seeps through the bandage, don't change it, just add more on top: dabbing a wound or changing a bandage removes any blood clot.

If blood is flowing with a pumping, squirting movement, an artery has been damaged. In this case medical help should be sought immediately,

but in the meantime continue to apply firm pressure. If you locate the local artery and press on it, this will be effective, but not for longer than 15 minutes at a time.

One exception: although scalp wounds bleed profusely, do not apply direct pressure if you suspect a skull fracture. Instead build up a dressing in the shape of a ring so that the pressure is applied around the wound, but not directly on it.

Cleaning wounds

Before you prepare to clean the wound, cover it with a clean cloth so that no more germs can enter it. Then wash your hands thoroughly, taking special care to scrub under the nails.

Wounds can be cleaned with a variety of liquids, from mild antiseptics to soap and water or mild detergents and water. Tap water is quite sterile, so it is not essential to boil water in a kettle.

If you use any antiseptic other than hydrogen peroxide, which is safe to use straight from the bottle, be sure to dilute it as instructed on the bottle. Using too strong a solution may damage the tissues and make the wound worse.

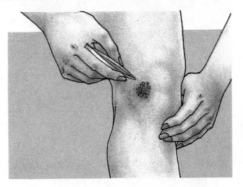

If there is any grit in the wound, a quick scrub with a clean brush under running water is an effective though painful way of removing it. Large pieces of grit and splinters should be removed individually with a pair of tweezers. If a large splinter will not lift out easily, it should be left until further medical care is given.

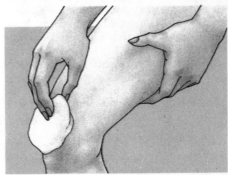

Brush any last bits of dirt from the surface of the wound with small swabs of gauze or cotton soaked in antiseptic. Then, working away from the wound, clean around it using fresh antiseptic swabs. Finally, clean the wound itself using separate swabs for every stroke. Work from the centre out.

Applying a dressing

A small, clean cut can be covered with adhesive bandages. These are specially prepared, thin strips of adhesive bandage used to hold the wound closed. The strips should be placed diagonally across each other, pulling the edges of the wound together.

A non-stick dressing is the best protection for a small wound as it can be removed without harming the scab. Never use cotton or the woolly side of lint as this sticks to the wound. Large wounds should be covered with sterile gauze dressings that take in the skin surrounding the wound as well.

Nigel Osborne

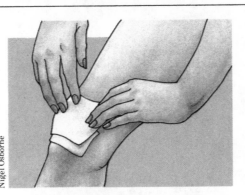

Then pad the dressing with cotton or additional layers of gauze: these will absorb any discharge and act as a protecting buffer. When the dressing is changed the layers should be peeled off individually.

Wrap the whole area firmly with a cotton or crepe bandage. Crepe is stretchy so it fits around awkward shapes easily. Dressings should be changed regularly. If the dressing has stuck to the wound, soak it off in a mild antiseptic solution. Never pull it off quickly as this will damage the scab.

Types of wound

There are five different types of wound: scratches, abrasions, cuts, lacerations and punctures. A scratch is a superficial tear through the outer layer of the skin called the epidermis. The edges of the skin are not separated and the small amount of bleeding comes from the tiny blood vessels within the skin itself. A scratch stops bleeding quickly but it is still a site for potential infection, especially if the skin is scratched by something dirty.

Abrasions

An abrasion is an area of skin that has been torn away by force. Light scuffing of the skin is called a graze, but sometimes a large, deep area of skin is affected and the abrasion is more like a severe burn. Occasionally an abrasion is so severe that a skin graft is needed some time later. Abrasions can be much more painful than cuts as millions of tiny nerve endings are exposed. They are nearly always full of dirt or grit, so the main problem is infection. After thoroughly cleaning the abrasion to remove dirt and grit, cover it with dry gauze until a scab forms.

Cuts

Any clean division through the layers of the skin is called a cut. Cuts are usually caused by sharp edges such as glass, razors, kitchen knives or even paper. They often bleed quite freely, especially if a deep cut damages large blood vessels underneath the skin, but this can usually be controlled.

Many cuts tend to gape slightly, so to aid the healing process keep the edges together with an adhesive bandage or porous synthetic surgical tape placed across the cut. This is especially advisable for cuts on the elbows or knees, which are constantly being bent, and on the fingers, which always seem to catch on something and so never stay closed long enough to heal.

If the cut gapes so badly that it cannot be held together with tape, or if it is deep enough to expose the layer of fat or muscle beneath the skin, it will need to be stitched. All cuts on the face, however minor, are best stitched to prevent scars.

Lacerations

A laceration is a tear in the skin and is usually caused by a hard blow or a serious injury. The skin edges are usually jagged, there is often considerable bruising around the wound, and infection is a particular hazard unless the wound is thoroughly cleaned.

Wounds of this sort will usually have to be seen by a doctor. They often bleed heavily and may be made worse by the

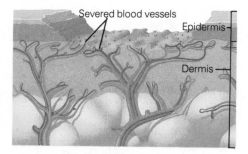

Abrasions are usually not as serious as they appear, though they may be very painful and leave scars afterwards. They must be thoroughly cleaned.

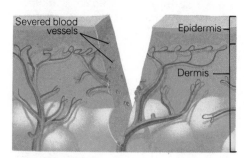

Cuts sometimes bleed profusely. They must be kept closed to heal properly and may need to be stitched, especially when they occur on the face.

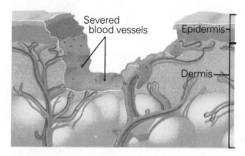

Lacerations are often serious wounds and take the longest time to heal. They should usually be seen by a doctor and kept covered meanwhile.

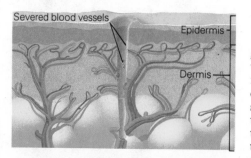

Puncture wounds are always more serious than they look, especially if to the abdomen or chest. Unless trivial, seek medical help as soon as possible.

presence of foreign objects like bullets large splinters embedded in them. Never attempt to pull these out. They have already done all the damage they are going to do and trying to remove them may start off massive bleeding. You can stop them from working deeper into the wound by building up a thick 'ring' dressing around them, but leave anything more to the doctor. Bandage all lacerations with a large dressing until a doctor can treat the wound.

Puncture wounds

Finally, a puncture or stab wound is a small, deep wound of unknown depth caused, for example, when the prong of a garden fork is run through the foot.

It is most important that you do not try to stop the bleeding—this is the only way the wound can clean itself. Once the bleeding has stopped on its own, wash the wound and apply a clean, dry dressing.

Except for those made by something small and clean like a thumbtack, all puncture wounds require medical attention as there is danger of internal bleeding, damage to tendons and nerves and increased chance of infection and tetanus, as tetanus germs thrive in deep closed wounds, where there is no oxygen. A good rule of thumb is that a puncture or stab wound is always worse than it looks, so be sure to seek help for anything more than the most negligible wounds.

What the doctor will do

Although usually minor wounds will not need any medical attention, especially if first aid is applied quickly, major wounds or very dirty ones will need to be looked at by a doctor.

The doctor will clean the wound thoroughly and explore it to ensure that there are no remaining foreign bodies. If there is any risk that splinters of glass or bits of metal are still in the wound, an X-ray may be taken. The doctor will then check that the nerves and tendons are functioning normally and will decide whether a tetanus injection is necessary and whether the wound needs stitching (suturing).

Stitches are used to pull the edges of a gaping wound together. This closes the wound to further contamination, makes it easier for the edges to join together and decreases the chances of an unsightly scar. However, stitches will not be used if the wound can be held closed without them as they can injure the surrounding tissue slightly and may leave additional scars. To get the best result, stitching if it is needed should be done as soon as possible. A local anaesthetic will usually be given to deaden the area surrounding the wound.

Recognizing and treating serious wounds

FIRST AID

Aside from the specific wounds that require a doctor's attention, there are a few obvious signs that indicate that medical attention is needed urgently. Ideally one person should apply first aid while a second calls for help. If you are alone you will have to assess each situation individually and decide what immediate first aid is necessary before calling for help. All the instances below require medical attention, but this may only become apparent after initial first aid has been applied. Lose no time in seeking help when needed—never feel you should try to cope alone.

Symptoms	Possible causes	Action
Bleeding persists	An artery may have been severed, in which case the blood will spurt out with each heart beat. Or there may be a deep puncture	Apply pressure in the normal way for at least ten minutes. If an artery is severed try to locate a 'pressure point', a place where a main artery can be pressed against a bone. Pressure can be applied at these points to stop arterial blood loss, but it should not be applied for any longer than 15 minutes without a break
Patient shows signs of shock. Usually all the following symptoms will be present: pale face and lips, cold and clammy skin, faint or dizzy feeling and weak and rapid pulse	Caused by a combination of low blood pressure, constriction of blood vessels and blood loss. The body diverts remaining blood to essential organs, such as kidney, heart and brain. If shock is combined with no visible sign of blood loss, there may be internal bleeding	Place patient comfortably on side and cover with blankets or clothing. If possible, raise the feet so that blood is concentrated in the area of vital organs. Loosen any tight clothing. It is important to reassure someone in shock, so stay by the person if possible. Never give the patient any liquids
Patient experiences loss of movement or tingling sensations in the wounded area	A tendon or nerve may be severed (tendons attach muscles to the bone at joints, such as the knee)	Apart from general first aid, there is no immediate treatment for this. Try not to move the patient while awaiting medical help

Healing

Healing begins very soon after injury. The white blood cells that rush to the site of the wound to clear infection also remove any cells that have died as a result of the injury, as well as the small quantities of blood that have collected around the wound.

Once the injury is clean, the healing process can begin under the protective covering of the scab. The remaining live skin cells divide rapidly and begin to produce fibrous scar tissue, which contains blood vessels and nerve fibres. The scar tissue grows up from the base of the wound, gradually filling the hole. When this process has finished, the scab will fall off.

The more quickly the surfaces of a wound are brought together, either by stitching or bandaging, the less fibrous tissue is produced to bind them. Healing is therefore quicker and the wound leaves a fainter scar.

Wounds that have been stitched become waterproof within 24 hours and generally heal within five days, when the stitches can be removed. Over the next few months, all the reddish scar tissue becomes white as it gets denser and loses blood vessels. As the scar tissue becomes denser it contracts, and this causes the puckering that is sometimes seen around large scars. If a scar is unsightly it can be improved by a skin graft. Scar tissue never grows hairs, doesn't have sweat glands and will not turn brown in the sun, but it is strong and protects the body just as well as the original skin.

TAKE CARE

Wounds that require a doctor's attention

● wounds that will not stop bleeding
● any very large, deep, gaping or jagged wounds
● any wounds where dirt or grit are embedded beneath the skin
● puncture wounds caused by anything dirty or rusty
● any cut on the face
● any wound that shows signs of infection.

Even when the greatest care is taken with a wound, there is always a danger of infection developing. Local infection in a wound is quite common and will produce a discharge of pus. If the wound is relatively minor, the infection will probably be dealt with by the body's natural defence mechanisms, but if the area around the wounds becomes very red and irritated, or the patient develops a fever, a doctor should be consulted as antibiotics may be needed.

Any pus that is formed should be allowed to drain off. If the infected wound has been stitched, it may be necessary to release some of the stitches. Infected abrasions should be bathed and freshly dressed each day.

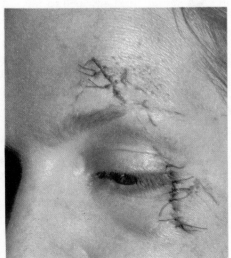

Ken Moreman

Q My son scraped his knee badly on a gravel path. I cleaned it carefully and washed all the little stones away with clean warm water and applied antibiotic ointment and clean dressing, but the wound became infected. What should I have done?

A The first aid treatment you administered was certainly sensible, but with an abrasion such as you describe tiny bits of gravel and dirt can easily get embedded in the tissue where they are hard to see and impossible to remove simply by washing the wound. In the case of serious abrasions, it is best to have the doctor examine the wound to decide on what treatment is necessary to prevent infection. Extreme care is necessary in applying antiseptic ointment as it should be borne in mind that a thick coating can seal in bacteria. Also, as with all home medical supplies the date of purchase should be checked. and any medication passed its use by date should be discarded. Only use cream for the purpose specified.

Q How long should I keep putting a new dressing on an abrasion?

A Once the wound has begun to heal, stop using any ointment and use a dry gauze dressing to keep the dirt out. Change the plain dressing when it gets grubby, and apply an antiseptic powder to the wound to help the scab to form if you wish.

Q Accident victims are sometimes described as having 'abrasions and contusions'. What is the difference?

A An abrasion is a wound in which the surface of the skin has been broken, so there will be some blood. A contusion, on the other hand, is a wound in which the surface of the skin is not broken; in other words, a bruise. People unfortunate enough to be involved in a car accident, for instance, can be slightly injured and have multiple scrapes and bruises. If you are ever called upon to administer first aid in such circumstances, remember that internal injuries are a real danger, as is shock.

This abrasion (right) on the calf of the leg has become infected. But if it is cleaned regularly with antiseptic or salt water solution, it will quickly heal.

A deep cut on a constantly moving joint like the knee (below), will take longer to heal and may leave a permanent scar.

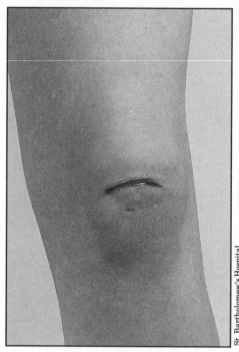

St. Bartholomew's Hospital

Healing difficulties

There are various complications that can arise from abrasions and cuts, and it is important to be aware of these and make regular checks as the healing process can be hindered by adverse conditions such as dirt, dampness or constant rubbing. The most important factor is thorough cleaning, even though this may be painful. Dirt embedded in tissue, and badly damaged tissue should be removed by a doctor as bacteria can breed and multiply on dead tissue. Antiseptic should only be applied to a clean wound as any antiseptic applied to a wound already contaminated will be ineffective since the dirt and germs will be pushed deeper into the wound.

Without thorough cleaning there is the possibility of invasion of the area by micro-organisms which will cause infection and produce a septic condition. The most obvious sign of a septic condition is pus, which is composed of tissue fragments, bacteria and dead white blood cells – these white cells being called to the area of inflammation to fight infection. Other signs of infection to watch out for are redness, which is a symptom of the dilation of blood vessels due to inflammation, soreness, swelling and increasing pain.

If infection does occur, treatment will depend on the severity of the condition, ranging from salt water bathing and poultices to antibiotics administered locally or orally. The point of infection may need to be opened and drained of pus by a doctor or trained medical staff.

Minor scratches and scrapes on the skin may invite Impetigo, a highly contagious infection of the outer layers of the skin resulting in weeping blisters. Treatment with antibiotics will be necessary combined with rigorous hygiene.

In view of these possible complications, it is essential to regularly check the healing progress. Any dressing that is wet or dirty should be removed and replaced, and, ideally, dressings should be removed once a dry scab has formed, though in certain cases, such as exposure to dirt or friction from clothing, some protection may be necessary.

If the abrasion or cut is in an area that is constantly moved, the knee, for example, it may be necessary to lubricate the area with ointment to prevent cracking.

The healing of abrasions and cuts is a good example of the body's ability to heal itself given the right conditions, freedom from infection, protection from rubbing and knocks and a good blood supply. Any scar left will continue to heal for 18 months and demonstrates the skin's ability to generate new tissue.

Abscess

Q How does all that pus get into an abscess?

A It doesn't actually 'get into' the abscess but builds up as part of the body's natural reaction to infection. Blood automatically rushes to the site of any injury, and when there is an infection the white blood cells, the body's infection-fighting team, move out of the damaged area into the infected tissue to kill the bacteria. In the struggle, the white blood cells often die themselves, and it is these dead cells, together with the dead bacteria, that form the well-known patch of yellow pus. At the same time, reserve forces of white blood cells build a wall that encloses the abscess's dangerous bacteria to keep the surrounding tissue intact and free from infection.

Q Why is an abscess in the ear so painful?

A Abscesses always involve considerable swelling. In the skin, this does not cause much discomfort, but in an area surrounded by bone, such as the ear, there is not enough space for this to happen without stretching the tissues around it, giving rise to great pain. For the same reason, severe discomfort accompanies any abscess in bone itself.

Q If I have an abscess on a tooth, must I have the tooth out?

A Not necessarily. If you seek treatment early enough, the dentist can open the gum to drain the pus until the infection subsides, and can also prescribe antibiotics to prevent the infection from spreading. But often the only way to release the pus is by pulling out the tooth.

Q What is a gumboil?

A If infection gets in between the tooth and gum, a relatively harmless abscess will form, ballooning out the gum until it bursts. This gumboil is different to a dental abscess caused by infection in the tooth socket. A hot, salty mouthwash may relieve discomfort and help to rupture the abscess so that the pus can drain away, but if the trouble persists, visit the dentist.

An abscess is the body's way of fighting localized infection. Minor abscesses often clear up with simple treatment, but larger or internal ones invariably need medical attention.

Abscesses can occur anywhere in, or on, the body. They range from simple styes, pimples and boils, which are abcesses in the skin's hair follicles, to serious tooth abscesses or other internal abscesses like an appendicitis.

Causes

All abscesses are caused by infection setting up inside a localized area of the body. Sometimes the entry point for infection is quite obvious: an abscess may occur, for example, as a result of a neglected injury to the skin or a large

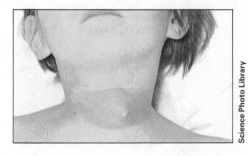

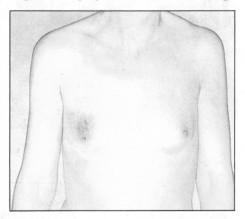

splinter. Often, however, there is no obvious site of entry for germs, but they can penetrate the skin through the microscopic pores in the skin surface. So if the skin is broken and dirty, abscesses are more likely.

Abscesses are also more common in moist areas of the body where there are larger pores in the skin, such as the armpit, groin and around the anus. Indeed, occasionally some people develop recurrent abscesses in these areas because the large glands which lie under the skin surface in time become deformed and persistently infected—a relatively rare condition called *Hydradenitis suppuritiva*.

Women who are breast-feeding sometimes develop a painful abscess in one

A serious abscess on the throat (top). Breast abscesses can occur at any time, but they are more common when a woman is breast feeding as germs can enter the milk duct through a cracked nipple.

The only safe way to drain a large, deep abscess is by surgical incision.

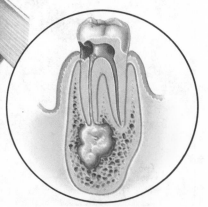

Gumboils develop when infection develops between the tooth and gum. More serious tooth abscesses (inset) develop in the tooth socket. In extreme cases the infection may be carried to the brain.

segment of the breast, as a result of infection gaining entry through a cracked nipple.

Some people do, at times, seem to be more prone to skin abscesses. Occasionally this is an early sign of lowered resistance to infection. Diabetes may be one possible cause: another is the presence of virulent bacteria on the skin surface—*Staphylococcus aureus*. These germs can live in moist, warm areas of the body, such as the nostrils, from where they are spread to other parts of the body by touch.

Internal abscesses are usually secondary to some other problem—a 'grumbling appendix' may be caused by an internal abscess formed because an intestinal blockage has irritated the appendix—although, as with an abscess caused by tuberculosis, the disease-causing bacteria may be breathed in or ingested via contaminated food.

Symptoms

The earliest sign of a skin abscess is a red, hot, painful swelling, which becomes filled with pus. If white blood cells are able to cope with the bacteria, the abscess clears up without any discharge, becoming a hard, painless lump which may disappear after some months.

Other symptoms, particularly of internal abscesses, are a fever and a feeling of being generally unwell. If the abscess is on the skin surface, glands nearby can become swollen and tender. So an abscess or boil on the arm can cause swollen glands in the armpit and one on the leg can cause swollen glands in the groin.

The great risk with an abscess is that on bursting it may release pus and dangerous live bacteria into the bloodstream, causing a serious type of blood-

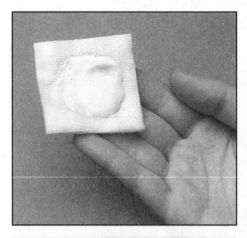
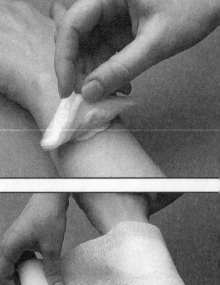
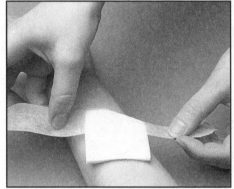

A poultice of magnesium sulphate is a simple and effective way of treating a small abscess. When applied hot, it softens the tissues and encourages it to rupture. Place the paste on gauze, place it on the abscess and bandage.

Staphylococcus bacteria (below) is commonly present on skin and mucous membranes and causes boils and internal abscesses. It is the commonest cause of pus-forming infections in man.

poisoning called septicaemia. A quickly rising fever will indicate that bacteria have entered the blood stream and this can be followed by a sudden lowering of blood pressure which will cause the patient to become pale and shocked. This condition is regarded as a medical emergency. In the case of an appendix abscess, pus and bacteria will be released into the abdominal cavity producing peritonitis (inflammation of the abdominal lining).

Treatment

Provided a skin abscess is treated at an early stage and the pus is drained safely away, it will cause little more than discomfort. A small superficial abscess will often discharge pus of its own accord—or, if obstinate, it can be 'lanced' with a sterile needle heated to red-hot and then allowed to cool.

Small abscesses can be drawn using a dry dressing covered with magnesium sulphate paste, which can be bought at any chemist: larger ones require medical attention. If the abscess is in an early stage of development antibiotics taken by mouth, or given by injection may cure the infection. Once any large quantity of pus has formed, the abscess may need to be drained by an incision made under local or general anaesthetic. Often antibiotics are needed to ensure that there is no danger of the infection spreading.

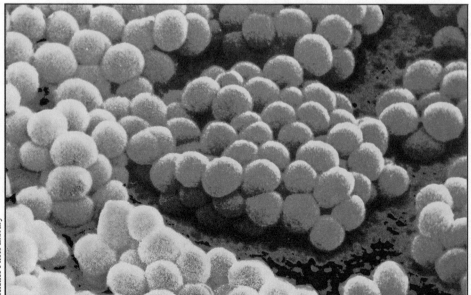

Accident prevention

Q **What can I do to help make sure that my children won't get injured at home?**

A First make a safe house—then get into the right safety habits. Here are some of the most important points to keep in mind. Make sure that you NEVER

● assume that visiting children have the same safety awareness as your own.

● allow children to play with sharp objects or run holding knives or scissors.

● permit games such as chasing on stairs or pushing wheeled toys into the kitchen.

● allow children to play with matches, lighters or cigarettes. Cigarette ends can poison a child.

● leave little ones in the bath alone.

● allow children to move electrical appliances alone, and never take any into the bathroom.

● leave baby alone with a bottle or young children with their meal. They could easily choke.

● allow young children to help with DIY jobs around the house.

● leave children alone with a hot iron while you go out of the room.

● keep medicines in your handbag. Never take them in front of the children or describe then as candy.

● keep your home medicines in the same place as household goods like rubbing alcohol so that the two could get confused.

● leave plastic bags or polyethylene wrappers where the children can reach them and suffocate themselves.

● leave your child alone in the house even for five minutes.

Q **Are there any particular times when my children are more likely to have accidents?**

A Illness, tiredness, lack of supervision and general family stress may all make your child more prone to accidents. Weekends, when more is going on in the home, are a particularly hazardous time. Many injuries to children occur when their parents are either out of the house or asleep. Drugs can also contribute, so if, for example, your child is taking antihistamines for an allergy be especially watchful, as these medicines cause drowsiness.

Every year a large number of children have accidents in the home. Sadly, many die of their injuries. But most home accidents could easily be prevented if parents were more aware of the hazards—and made sure their home was safe for children.

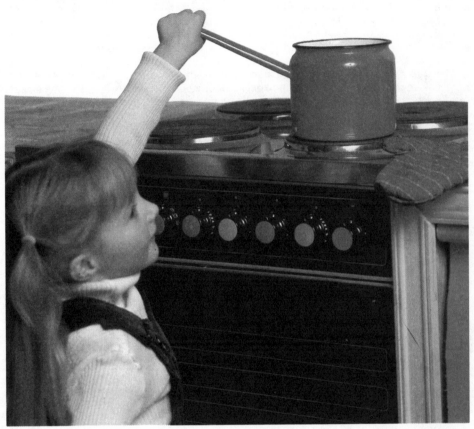

Di Lewis

Safety in the home is of the greatest importance for the well-being of children and parents alike. Recognizing the risks in the first place, and then taking adequate measures to ensure that your children are not in any danger is a vital part of responsible parenthood and will relieve you of much anxiety.

It is sensible to start making your home safe *before* you have a family so that when your children are born they start life in the best possible situation.

Preparing a safe home
If you are expecting a baby, start by drawing up a checklist of home safety measures you can carry out immediately. This should include making (or buying) safety gates for stairs, kitchen and outside doors; fixing loose rugs firmly to floors to avoid them causing falls; installing dummy plugs in any unused electric wall sockets; keeping dangerous household equipment out of children's reach—knives, can openers, cleaning powders; investing in safe heaters and fireguards;

and ensuring that the home is well lit.

Next, learn safety habits yourself so that you will automatically follow them by the time you have children.

Lock away all medicines, including contraceptive pills and creams, indigestion tablets and iron and vitamin pills. Start running cold water before hot into the bath to avoid any danger of scalding at bathtime. Test out your furniture to discover which tables and chairs are least likely to topple over.

Take great care with fire and be especially careful in the kitchen, which is second only to the living/dining room as the most dangerous area in the house. If you do have a fire and cannot put it out easily, call the fire brigade. Make sure your older children know how to do this and keep your doctor's number by the telephone too.

Smooth areas of flooring in kitchens and bathrooms need non-slip surfaces like cork tiles, and liquid spills, especially of soap, cooking oil or other grease should be wiped up at once.

Day-to-day safety care

One of the commonest causes of death among the under-4s is suffocation—normally by choking on food—and the major cause of all hospital admissions for children under 14 is poisoning, either by medicines or by household substances. Among the 5s to 14s many deaths are from burns, while little ones aged one to two are vulnerable to all home accidents.

With a demanding baby, a safe daily routine will help when you are tired and preoccupied. Always put the things you use back in a safe place and do not use too much of anything—even talcum powder can cause choking. Be very watchful at bathtime. Do not be tempted to overfeed a baby, but if a baby does choke, keep calm and slap it between the shoulder blades to clear the air passages. After feeding always take the baby's bib off. Buy a cat net for the pram as cats are fond of seeking warmth from babies' blankets.

At the toddler stage—when children need particularly careful supervision—try to hear anything you cannot actually see, and beware of silence!

Clearly it is essential to supervise all meals. Spend time teaching your children how to climb stairs—they cause more accidents in the home than any other household objects—and show them how to balance and jump correctly from them. Help little ones to understand about hot and cold food and water, and show them how to carry breakable objects safely. Finally, to keep yourself alert, try to take some time off and hand the children over to someone you trust while staying on call should you be needed. The only common pets that are potentially dangerous are dogs. They should be obedience trained and never left alone with any child.

Children need careful supervision in the home, but at the same time it is important to allow them enough freedom to learn to deal independently and safely with their home environment.

Safe for children

Equipment bought especially for children is high on the danger list, but properly chosen, used and maintained it can be safe.

Prams should not tip over easily and should have an attachment for a safety harness. The brake should not be within the baby's reach and should work well even if the pram is tipped forward.

Folding pushchairs should have two sets of locking devices and so should the handle if this folds separately. Neither pushchairs nor prams can work properly if they are overloaded with other children or shopping.

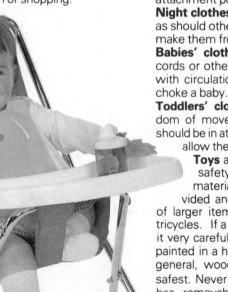

Car beds and travelling cribs should be sturdy and not easily tipped, and the handles should ensure a safe ride when the bed is carried by two people. If a crib is collapsible, it must not be likely to collapse accidentally. Ensure that the crib and stand are made of harmless rustproof material.

High chairs must be without sharp ends, open tubes where small limbs might get caught, or mechanisms that could pinch. The chair should not move on castors. Buy one that is at a convenient height, is sturdy, and has attachment points for a safety harness.

Night clothes must be flame-resistant, as should other clothes or the fabric you make them from.

Babies' clothes should be free from cords or other ties, which can interfere with circulation or could even hang or choke a baby.

Toddlers' clothes should allow freedom of movement and growth. They should be in at least part-natural fabric to allow the skin to breathe.

Toys are subject to government safety regulations in terms of materials used, instructions provided and the design and stability of larger items like baby walkers and tricycles. If a toy is secondhand, check it very carefully; some old toys were painted in a highly toxic lead paint. In general, wooden and plastic toys are safest. Never give a baby any toy that has removable buttons or bits that might be swallowed. All toys should be easy to clean.

Keep a safe home

Child's room

Keep small toys out of the way, to be used under supervision

Fit safety locks and/or bars (removable in case of fire) to all windows so that children cannot open them more than 2 in

Use a toy basket that will not squeeze fingers if the lid slams shut

Make sure bars of bed or crib are not more than 2½ in apart

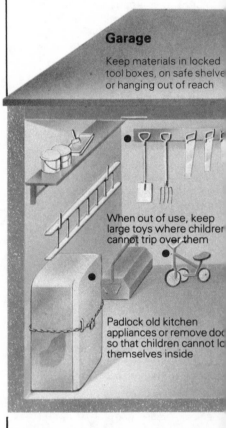

Garage

Keep materials in locked tool boxes, on safe shelves or hanging out of reach

When out of use, keep large toys where children cannot trip over them

Padlock old kitchen appliances or remove doors so that children cannot lock themselves inside

Child's room

Beds and cribs should be solid and smooth with no sharp projections inside and no horizontal bars, which could help a child climb out. Any dropside mechanism should fasten automatically so that the child cannot loosen it.

A convector heater is the safest way to heat a child's room

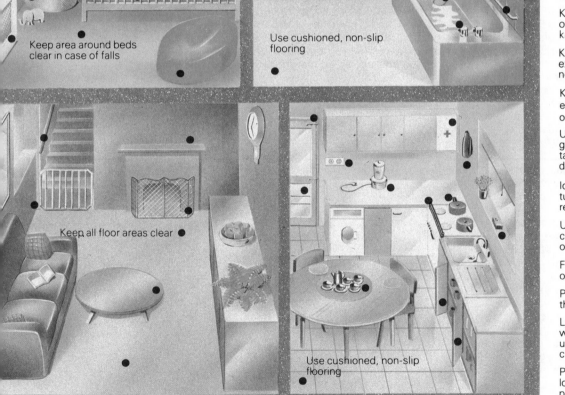

Bathroom

Electric heaters should be wall or ceiling mounted, with a pull switch at adult height

Lock all medicines in a cupboard. Put aerosols, razors and cosmetics in a high cupboard

Dry or air clothes over towel rails only

Radiators should not be too hot to touch. Keep hot water tank set at medium

Use large, preferably plastic bath toys

A hand grip and rubber mat prevent falls

Kitchen

Fit bolts to all doors that only adults can reach

Put matches well out of child's reach. Choose gas cooker without a pilot light and use an electric lighter

Keep a locked first aid box or cupboard to hand in kitchen

Keep a small fire extinguisher or heavy cloth near cooker to put out fires

Keep toaster and other equipment out of reach, on a short electric cord

Use tempered or laminated glass in doors, marked with tape or transfers so children don't walk into it

Ideally, fit a pan guard, or turn handles back out of reach

Use table mats instead of cloths. Keep hot drinks out of reach

Fit dummy plugs or covers on risky sockets

Put heavy items where they cannot fall on children

Leave only safe-to-play-with equipment in an unlocked floor-level cupboard

Put household cleaners in a locked cupboard or in a high place. Make sure they are clearly marked

Image labels:

Fit locks that can be worked from inside and out

Keep area around beds clear in case of falls

Use cushioned, non-slip flooring

Keep all floor areas clear

Use cushioned, non-slip flooring

---

se absorbent cotton bed sheets (never [pl]astic). Sheets should be fitted or lightly [tu]cked in

[C]hildren's furniture should be soft, low and [fr]ee from sharp edges, and positioned so that [th]ey cannot climb onto shelves or window [si]lls

[T]o prevent suffocation, use a porous type [pi]llow, or none at all for babies under 1 year. [P]illow cases should be cotton and well fitted

Living room

Fit a hand rail. Keep stairs well lit and free from ill-fitting carpets or jumble

An open fire must be fitted with a fixed guard. Position an extra one far enough away so that the bars do not get hot

Keep area over fire clear to avoid attracting a child's attention

Use safety gates, at top and bottom of stairs, at kitchen doors and other potentially dangerous places

Make sure all furniture and fitments are secure and will support a child's weight

Ideally, fit a hard-wearing carpet except in kitchen and bathroom. Alternatively, fix any loose rugs to prevent slips. Do not lay rugs on polished floors.

Acne

Q Does acne always leave scars on the skin?

A No, but the chances of scarring are increased if you pick and squeeze the spots. However, even if the blackheads are not squeezed, scars may still form. If they are severe they can be partially removed by a minor surgical operation called dermabrasion, in which the top layers of skin are rubbed away, leaving the skin relatively smooth.

Q My daughter has very bad acne. Should I take her to the doctor?

A Yes. The doctor can prescribe antibiotics over a period of several months to reduce secondary infection of the spots by bacteria, or may put her on the birth control Pill, which contains hormones that help correct the hormone imbalance that causes acne. And the reassurance and advice about hygiene the doctor gives may well be easier for your daughter to accept as it comes from someone outside the family circle.

Q Is it true that chocolate causes acne?

A Acne has several causes that are not necessarily connected with diet. It is was once thought that cutting out chocolate would help it clear up more quickly and stop new spots forming. There is no certainty, however, that chocolate is the culprit but if you have acne, it may be worth dropping it from your diet for a while to see whether it makes any difference. There are several other foods which sometimes affect acne, and your doctor may suggest that you try avoiding them too. On the positive side, he may suggest you eat lots of fresh fruit and vegetables and drink plenty of water.

Q I get the occasional spot. Is this acne?

A No, acne is a whole mass of blackheads and pimples. The odd spot can also be caused by a hormone imbalance, as before a period, but it is just as likely that an unhealthy diet, poor hygiene or being run down is to blame.

The pimpled face of adolescence is so common that it could almost be thought of as normal. Four out of five teenagers suffer from acne to some degree, but the majority grow out of it. In the meantime, there are preventive measures and treatments which can ease the problem.

The mixture of blackheads, whiteheads and pink or reddish spots caused by *Acne vulgaris* occurs mostly on the face, the back of the neck, the upper back and chest, but can sometimes be found in the armpits and on the buttocks, too.

Causes

Acne affects young people of both sexes but tends to be more common in boys. It starts in adolescence because this is when there are great increases in the production of hormones from the sex organs and from the adrenal glands. These hormones are chemical messengers carried by the blood and transform a child into a sexually mature adult.

Under their influence, and particularly that of the androgens, or 'masculinizing' hormones, the oil-releasing sebaceous glands in the skin, which normally produce just enough oil or sebum to keep the skin healthily supple, become over active. They release too much sebum causing a condition called *seborrhoea*.

The female hormones, particularly oestrogen, have the reverse effect, which explains—at least in part—why girls are generally less prone to acne than boys.

Symptoms

Blackheads, accompanied by the pink or reddish inflammation which they cause are the hallmark of acne. It was once thought that the bacteria that naturally thrive on sebum, particularly two called *Staphylococcus albus* and *Bacillus acnus* were the underlying cause of the acne

How to alleviate the symptoms of acne

AVOID
- greasy hair oils or cosmetics.
- leaving makeup on overnight—or leave it off completely
- applying creams to dirty skin so that bacteria are pushed into the pores
- eating any foods that seem to cause spots

TRY TO
- wash affected areas several times a day with soap and hot water
- wash hair often wear it off the face and reasonably short
- keep combs, brushes and washcloths clean and grease-free
- get as much sunshine as you possibly can

Di Lewis

18

t they are now known to be the cause of e inflammation, not the acne itself.

In response to the presence of bacteria, hich multiply in the blackhead, the ood vessels expand to bring more infction-fighting cells to the site—this is e inflammatory reaction. As a seconary effect of acne, the bacterial infection ay lead to the development of pimples, hich are spots filled with dead white lls and bacteria, or pus.

This infection usually only becomes vere, involving the formation of larger ils or abscesses, if the deeper skin ssues become bruised and damage as a sult of squeezing the blackheads to lease the core of sebum plugged in the re. Left undisturbed, each spot or ackhead usually clears up within about week, but if secondary infection sets in may take a month or more.

angers

econdary infection is one of the chief ysical dangers of acne, as it can lead to vere permanent scars and crater-like ts of pock-marks in the complexion. ven more severe is the psychological nger, for acne can turn a happy exovert into a morose introvert. So anye suffering from acne needs all the assurance possible to prevent a tempory physical problem from becoming one at is psychologically permanent.

Try to take a practical approach to eatment and dispel any fears engenered by old wives' tales—for example, at acne is caused by masturbation or xual intercourse.

reatment

n a day-to-day basis, the most impornt treatment is washing. This is most fective if it is as vigorous as possible,

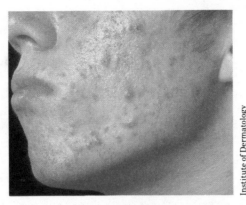

Institute of Dermatology

and a soft nailbrush or loofah—kept scrupulously clean to avoid reinfection— will help to remove grease and encourage the top layer of skin to peel away, taking with it some, if not all, of the plug of sebum. Drying, equally vigorously, with a rough, clean towel will have the same effect. An astringent cleansing lotion applied with clean cotton after thorough washing will help to remove any remaining oil.

It is possible to remove the blackheads with an instrument called a comedone extractor. However, this must be used with great care, preferably only on the recommendation of a doctor, and with meticulous attention to hygiene, to prevent the possibility of secondary infection.

A clean face will be of little help to the acne problem if it is then surrounded by lank, greasy hair. Unfortunately the overactivity of the sebaceous glands is not confined to the face but also affects the scalp, and the hair tends to become excessively greasy with the usual associated development of scurf or dandruff. The grease from the hair aggravates the acne, so hair should be washed regularly and kept reasonably short.

Creams and lotions can be useful to treat acne, as much for their camouflage effect as for medical reasons. The best preparations are those that contain substances such as calamine, zinc sulphate, sulphur, resorcinol or benzoyl peroxide, which tend to dry the skin and cause peeling of the top layer. Boys may regard such creams as an insult to their masculinity, but many modern ones are very natural-looking and may prove a very useful psychological prop.

A well balanced diet containing plenty of fresh fruit and vegetables is always good for the skin, and the acne sufferer is advised to drink a lot of water to keep the circulation well flushed of the toxins that are likely to aggravate the condition.

Many acne sufferers find that pimples clear up more quickly in summer. This is because the ultra-violet light in sunshine helps dry up grease on the skin and aids peeling of the top layer. For the same reason, ultra-violet ray lamps are often advised for acne sufferers, but these should be used with care to prevent the skin burning.

It is always sensible for a teenager with very bad acne to see a doctor, who may be able to prescribe stronger treatment, such as tetracycline or retinoic acid.

Outlook

The best that can be said for acne is that it does not last forever. Usually there is only one really bad year, and acne is rare after the mid-twenties. Difficult though it may be to follow, the best advice is to resist with a will of iron the temptation to pick and squeeze blackheads.

Finally, keep a look out for new treatments, such as preparations containing retinoic acid, which have shown encouraging results in clinical trials.

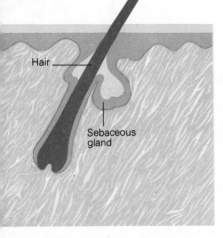

acne, extra sebum (oil) first clogs the pores through which sebum is leased to the skin surface.

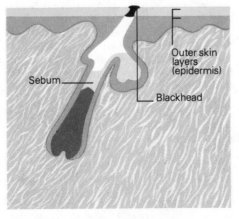

The sebum is trapped and forms a plug with a raised top which, when exposed to air, becomes a blackhead.

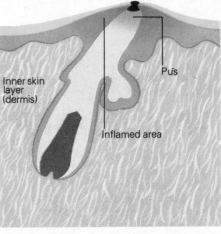

The surrounding skin then becomes inflamed and infected, resulting in pimples filled with pus.

Nigel Osborne

Acupuncture

Q Will acupuncture help me to stop smoking?

A Only if you really want to stop. It will help by reducing the withdrawal symptoms and the craving.

Q I've seen pictures of people with acupuncture needles in them. It looks as though it might be painful.

A Most people experience very little discomfort. There is a slight, brief prick as the needle enters the skin, but as the treatment takes effect there is usually a feeling of numbness, aching, swelling or tingling.

Q Does the insertion of the needles make you bleed?

A Usually no, because the smooth, fine and supple needles do not damage the tissues. Points on the ear and face bleed occasionally as the skin here has a rich blood supply.

Q How long does the treatment take to work?

A This depends on several factors. Acute complaints may improve immediately or within a week or two. Chronic conditions will take longer, perhaps two or three months of weekly treatments, although some benefit should be noticed within a few weeks.

Q Do I need a referral from my doctor before visiting an acupuncturist?

A A referral is not necessary, although it is always appreciated. If there is a good reason for you not to have acupuncture, your doctor will explain this to you.

Q Can people of all ages receive acupuncture?

A As a rough guide, anyone between the ages of 7 and 70 can receive acupuncture. If a child is not afraid of needle pricks and can remain still then there should be no problem. With older patients, moxibustion is often preferred to needle treatment.

Cure-all or con trick? Today, an increasing number of people are turning to acupuncture, and though not a miracle remedy, it does offer an alternative method of relieving pain and modern stress-related complaints.

Acupuncture is an ancient healing art that has been used in China for several thousand years. Following the discovery of acupuncture anaesthesia in China during the 1950s, several groups of Western doctors visited China to report on the technique. They were impressed, and interest in acupuncture grew rapidly with many of the techniques being incorporated into Western medical practice. Although often regarded as an alternative medicine, it has been surprisingly successful in the treatment of many ailments where more conventional methods have failed.

Perhaps the failure of acupuncture to become fully integrated with Western medical practice is due to the great difference between the cultures of the East and West. In ancient China, the emphasis was on preventative medicine, something which is relatively new in Western medical thought. It is this cultural division that has produced two explanations of how acupuncture works.

The Chinese origins

Acupuncture has its roots in the ancient Chinese philosophy of Taoism, where it was believed that man is one with the universe and that all life is permeated with the life-giving energy of Chi. Part of this belief is that all our experiences have opposites (hot/cold, day/night, masculine/feminine). Yin and Yang are the names given to these opposite forces.

The theory is that Yin and Yang merge and complement one another, creating a balance. When the forces are balanced we are in good health. However, when the flow is out of balance within ourselves and with the universe we feel unwell and disease may develop.

Acupuncture is used to restore the balance, the acupuncture points being the places where treatment is applied. These acupuncture points lie above lines under the skin called meridians, and the ancient theorists believed these lines acted as channels through which the Yin and Yang energies flowed. Whether one is sympathetic to this theory or not, acupuncture worked for the ancient Chinese.

Modern theory

Today, Western practitioners of acupuncture explain its effectiveness in more scientific terms, though still incorporating some of the Oriental beliefs.

Frank Kennard

Meridian lines

Lung · Kidney · Heart · Stomach · Spleen

Their explanation is based on Western knowledge of the body's nervous system.

Beneath the skin is a widespread network of nerves, the most important strands of which run along the meridians where most acupuncture points lie.

Among their functions, the nerves pass on messages that take the form of feelings which tell us what state our bodies are in. These messages come from all over the body and when they arrive from a damaged organ an 'alarm' sounds at the

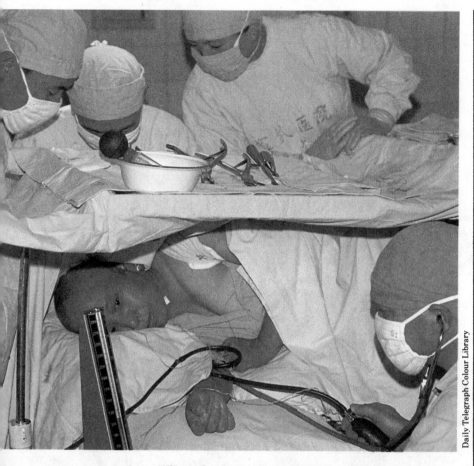

Daily Telegraph Colour Library

> **What acupuncture can and cannot do**
>
> Acupuncture has proved helpful in the treatment of a number of different problems, both physical and mental. But it is not a cure-all.
>
> **IT CAN**
> - alleviate the symptoms of stress: headaches, anxiety, tension, insomnia
> - relieve pain, and can be used as an anaesthetic
> - improve many rheumatic complaints such as lumbago, sciatica, and certain types of arthritis
> - aid respiratory problems, such as asthma, bronchitis, coughs
> - help digestive problems such as ulcers, nausea, colitis
> - benefit those with sex-related problems, such as period pains and impotence
> - aid the treatment of heart complaints, high or low blood pressure, eye and skin problems, among many others.
>
> **IT CANNOT**
> - cure cancer, mend broken bones or repair damaged tissue or organs
> - remove the root causes of complaints, and may sometimes disguise them
> - always work on its own.
>
> For instance, the cure for stress and tension may be effective only if accompanied by changes in diet and lifestyle.

erve endings in the skin. When this appens the alarm is felt as pain. The heory is that the pain may be referred; hat is, it may be a signal of a problem ocated elsewhere in the body rather than here the pain is felt.

For instance, pain from the stomach is egistered in the skin of the upper abdomen and the adjacent part of the back. he connection between the source of the roblem and where the pain is felt is explained by the fact that both areas have nterconnecting nerves.

There are a thousand or so acupuncture oints in the body dotted along the eridian lines. There are 12 main meridians and each is associated with an rgan of the body. The lines run along the ajor parts of the body (such as the arms nd legs) and end at the tips of the fingers r the toes. For instance, the liver eridian runs down the inside of the left g, from the midriff to the big toe.

ow it works

lthough the ancient Chinese believed at it was the rebalancing of Yin and ang energies that brought relief, odern scientific studies have indicated at there are at least two alternative eories.

The 'gate theory' is that there are reflex echanisms in the nerve pathways

Acupuncture needles can be inserted in any of the thousand or so points along the meridian lines. The needles have an anaesthetic effect powerful enough to allow brain surgery to take place with the patient fully conscious.

which can close off pain, rather as if a gate were being closed. This reduces the pain although the cause persists. Acupuncture works by closing these gates.

The other theory explains the success of acupuncture through the production of hormones called endorphins. These have a pain-killing effect, much like the drug morphine. There is now evidence that acupuncture causes the release of endorphins and these then travel to the brain, where they activate a mechanism which blocks the pain messages.

This theory helps to explain the pain-relieving effects of acupuncture and its ability to induce relaxation and a sense of well-being. However, no theory as yet manages to explain some of the claims of wonder cures.

The benefits of acupuncture

Acupuncture can be used to help with a wide range of specific problems, not just the relief of pain. These include headaches, rheumatic pains, digestive disorders, asthma, hypertension, insomnia,

anxiety, menstrual disorders and infertility. It is also used in childbirth and even in open-heart operations.

The treatment also gives a feeling of well-being and relaxation. For this reason it is an appropriate treatment or preventive for the numerous ailments caused by stress in our high-speed society. But acupuncture is not a cure-all. It is not appropriate for anyone who is at risk from infection (i.e. severe diabetics or people taking steroids), nor for those who have bleeding disorders such as haemophilia.

Treatment

The patient is questioned about his complaint and asked whether diet, mood, personal habits, season and weather have any effect on the problem.

A thorough physical examination then takes place, with the acupuncturist taking particular note of any tender areas, the pulse rate at the wrist, signs of tension, and variations in body temperature. Further information is sometimes obtained from examining the tongue, iris, and soles of the feet.

ACUPUNCTURE

For pain relief in childbirth, needles may be inserted in the toe, earlobe and hand. Those in the hand may be electrically stimulated according to the strength of the contractions. Only a slight tingling sensation is felt.

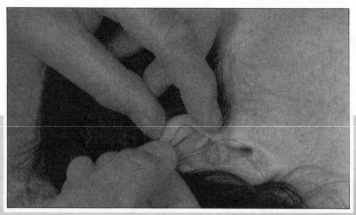

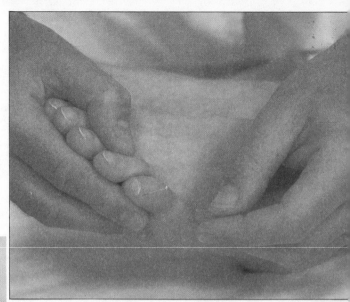

On the basis of all this information a diagnosis can be made, either in terms of diseases or of the classical concepts of Chi energy balance. The treatment then consists of applying needles, massage or heat to certain points on the body.

The heat treatment is called moxibustion because it involves placing rolled-up cones of the herb moxa on the correct meridian points and igniting them. A beneficial warmth is produced by their slow burning and the acupuncturist removes them before the skin is reached. Heat treatment can also be provided by electrical means, using a recent Japanese invention, but acupuncturists generally consider that it is no substitute for the original method.

The choice of the points depends on the condition of the patient; it will vary from person to person and from day to day as the condition changes. The number of needles used also changes; from one to 20 or more, and they may stay in for as long as the acupuncturist deems necessary.

The success of the treatment depends on many factors, among them diet and lifestyle.

One risk involved is that acupuncture applied thoughtlessly might hide a serious illness by taking away the symptoms. This is the reason for the very thorough examination and diagnosis.

A common response to the treatment is that the patients become so relaxed that they temporarily lose co-ordination after a session. For this reason, alcohol a[n]d sedatives should not be combined wi[th] acupuncture. Driving is also unwis[e] especially after the first session.

Treatment at home

Some acupuncture techniques can [be] learnt and practised at home. Th[is] applies more to acupressure, which is [a] form of massage acupuncture witho[ut] needles. It will provide relief fro[m] headaches, tension and anxiety, amo[ng] other stress complaints, and is perfect[ly] safe. The use of acupuncture is growi[ng] rapidly. There are now many colleg[es] that provide training in acupuncture a[nd] acupressure for those who wish to beco[me] qualified practitioners.

Adenoids

Q My child breathes through his mouth a lot. Does this mean he has adenoid trouble?

A Not necessarily. But if he also has nasal discharge and a night-time cough, adenoids are probably the cause. Otherwise it may be a habit, and is best cured by regular noseblowing. You should check his ability to breathe through each nostril in turn to make sure that something lodged in the nose is not the cause. A few children are born with bone abnormalities which prevent normal nose-breathing.

Q Can adenoids be diagnosed just by looking at a child's face?

A No. So-called 'adenoidal faces' have been found to occur in many other conditions. The description refers to a snub nose, high arched palate and protruberant upper teeth, which give the child a rather dopey look.

Q If my child has had his adenoids operated on can they regrow?

A Yes. They can regrow because it is surgically impossible to remove the whole of the glands. They are merely cut off as low as possible. This leaves a small stump which can enlarge again. However, as the stimulus to grow disappears around the age of six, regrowth does not usually cause problems.

Q How long is it safe to use decongestant nosedrops?

A Any runny nose will be dried up by decongestant drops. The problem is that if the cause has not been dealt with, stopping the drops will cause the discharge to return. In the case of adenoids, the problem for which they are needed will probably have improved after a week or so, and they should be stopped then. A slight discharge may return for a day or two, which will have to be tolerated without restarting the drops. If the drops are used for more than three weeks continually, there is a definite risk that the nose will counterbalance their effect by running all the time. And prolonged use can cause serious damage.

The adenoids have been called 'the watchdogs of the throat'. Like the tonsils, they guard against respiratory infection in the young child, but like the tonsils they sometimes become infected and swollen themselves.

Adenoids are lymph glands situated at the back of the nose just where the air passages join those of the back of the mouth or pharynx. The lymph system is the body's defence against infection and the lymph glands, such as the adenoids, are full of infection-fighting cells, the white blood cells. The adenoids are so placed that any infection breathed in through the nose is filtered by them and—hopefully—killed. Sometimes, however, things can go wrong.

Causes

Adenoids are present from birth, but on the whole they disappear before puberty. They are most obvious from the age of one to four. This is because between these ages the child is continually exposed to new types of infection.

Not a great deal is known about how the adenoids become infected, but any respiratory germ can affect them. Once they become damaged, chronic infection may set in. If the adenoids are recurrently inflamed, they tend to swell and this can give rise to ill-effects.

Symptoms

If the glands become swollen due to infection, they interfere with the flow of air through the nose so that the child has to breathe through the mouth. This may cause heavy snoring at night. The closed mouth also causes a nasal tone of speech. The child finds that his 'm' comes out as 'b' and 'n' sounds like 'd'. This is because when he closes his mouth to pronounce 'm' and 'n' through the nose, he cannot do so since his nose is blocked. Breathing

Inflamed and swollen adenoids can block the Eustachian tubes and lead to ear infections and even deafness.

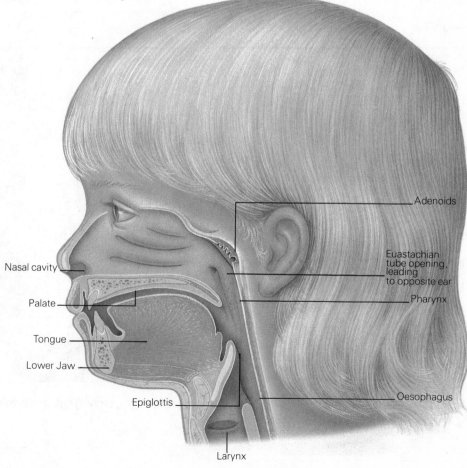

Nasal cavity

Palate

Tongue

Lower Jaw

Epiglottis

Larynx

Adenoids

Euastachian tube opening, leading to opposite ear

Pharynx

Oesophagus

Mike Courteney

Q Is sneezing and a runny nose due to adenoids?

A Usually not. These symptoms are more suggestive of an allergic nose problem. As research continues, many childhood illnesses are being found to be due to allergies. Often these are caused by dusts and pollens, and sneezing or a runny nose is their most obvious symptom. The medical treatment with decongestants and antihistamines is the same, but adenoidectomy would make no difference.

Q Is there a link between adenoids and mental deficiency?

A Certainly not! Though children with an adenoid problem may look dull and be slow to respond, careful studies have failed to show any such link. However, if left completely untreated, the complication of deafness can certainly prevent a child from realizing his true potential.

Q My child snores heavily. Could he have adenoids?

A Snoring can certainly be due to enlarged adenoids, but by itself this symptom does not need treating. Otherwise, snoring could be caused by an abnormality of the facial structure which the child probably had since birth. Many children breathe noisily at night, which is not true snoring but just a result of a catarrhal complaint such as the common cold.

Q Can antihistamines and antibiotics do anything to help treat adenoids?

A Antihistamines reduce the swelling of the adenoids when this has been caused by an allergic reaction as opposed to infection, and they will also tend to reduce the discharge as well. A further benefit is that antihistamines usually cause drowsiness and combat nausea so a bedtime dose will reduce coughing and the morning vomiting.

Antibiotics are of benefit for enlarged adenoids only when there is also a bacterial infection and must be prescribed by your doctor. The adenoidal symptoms may remain but painful complications such as ear infections can be prevented.

through the mouth also makes it very dry and the child may continually ask for something to drink.

As the adenoids fight infection, white blood cells—both dead and alive—are released in the form of pus. This pus will be seen as a discharge from the nose—quite different from the clear, watery discharge of a runny cold. The child sniffs to try to clear it but it then runs down the back of his throat and makes him cough. The cough is particularly obvious at night and is a typical sign of infected adenoids. In the morning, the swallowed pus may cause vomiting.

Dangers

Swollen adenoids can block the Eustachian tubes, which are a pair of tunnels running through the skull bones from inside each eardrum to the pharynx. Their function is to equalize the pressure in the middle ears with that outside—they give rise to the familiar 'pop' you hear on swallowing. If the tube is blocked by the enlarged adenoids the pressure cannot be balanced.

But the main hazard is that natural secretions in the ear cannot drain from inside. This gives rise to a 'glue ear' in which the hearing apparatus is stuck up by secretions and hearing is impaired.

And the secretions themselves ma[y] become infected causing a conditi[on] called *otitis media*. This is painful a[nd] can affect the hearing permanently. [If] untreated, the eardrums will usual[ly] burst to release the infection.

Treatment

Gargling is useless, but three types [of] medicines are helpful in treati[ng] adenoids. Decongestants and antih[is]tamines are on sale at the drugstore, b[ut] consult your doctor before using ther[m.] Antibiotics are available on prescripti[on.]

As a last resort, when other metho[ds] have failed, the adenoids may be remov[ed] by an operation called an adenoidectom[y.] The operation is fairly simple and [is] carried out under a general anaesthet[ic] in hospital. The tonsils are often remov[ed] in the same operation.

Outlook

Providing none of the serious comp[li]cations occur, time, the decline of infec[ti]ous diseases and improvements in trea[t]ment all mean that adenoids are not t[he] problem they were twenty years ag[o.] Often symptoms go away of their ov[wn] accord when the child is six or so, a[nd] modern medicines usually save sma[ll] children from an operation.

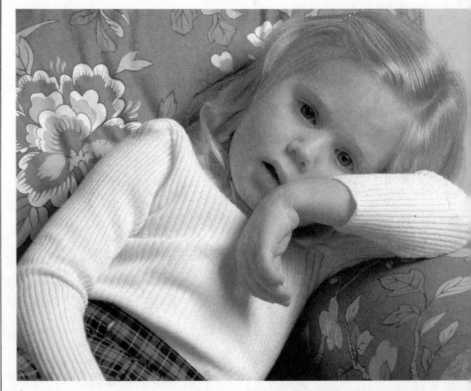

Some common symptoms of swollen adenoids

- hearing difficulties
- dry gums, which result in tooth decay, and halitosis

- loss of smell, taste and appetite
- listless expression, because breathing [is] such hard work

Adolescence

Q We used to have a very close relationship with our son. Now he has turned completely against us. Where did we go wrong?

A Nowhere. It is often the case that the closer the relationship, the more sudden the rebellion in adolescence. Just remember that this does not mean rejection. A child who storms at his or her parents still obviously cares what they think—more so probably than a child who simply ignores them.

Q Our 16-year-old daughter wants to go on the Pill, although she swears she is not sleeping with anyone. She says it is 'just in case'. Should I let her?

A Although you may be worried, the fact that she has consulted you is a compliment to your relationship with her. But do not forbid her to go on the Pill; she could consult a doctor and it would be prescribed if it was thought that she was sufficiently mature and responsible. You would not be told because medical matters are always confidential. Remember also that preventing her from going on the Pill will not stop her from having sexual relationships. So be realistic—she could come to you in a couple of months' time wanting not the Pill but an abortion. Or not coming to you at all, which would be worse.

Talk to her calmly and sympathetically. Point out that the Pill is a drug which should not be taken unnecessarily. Tell her what you feel, but remember that she needs to make her own decision once she is armed with a range of opinions and as much factual information as possible.

Q My 15-year-old son is terribly rude to me and my husband, but I'm afraid if I put my foot down it will turn him against us.

A Do put your foot down—firmly In the long run, he'll respect you for it, and that means you'll be doing him a favour: children who have no regard for their parents often never develop any self-respect themselves.

In adolescence young people are undergoing the physical and mental changes that take them into adulthood, and this can be a difficult time for them. It is vital that parents show sympathy and understanding—and are able to judge when professional help is needed.

Adolescence begins with the onset of puberty, when the body begins to develop rapidly. Boys quickly grow taller and more muscular at an amazing speed. Girls, too, increase rapidly in height; body fat begins to be redistributed to breasts, buttocks, hips and thighs and the menstrual periods start. In boys, the penis and testicles grow larger. Both sexes develop body hair in the armpits, the groin and on the limbs; boys begin to grow facial hair.

These changes are brought about by a complex interplay of hormones, or 'chemical messengers'—which are released into the bloodstream by the glands. Their effect is not only physical but also mental and emotional.

On average, adolescence starts around the age of 11 for girls and 13 for boys, but it can in fact begin at any time from 10 to 16 in both sexes.

A time of conflict

Before adolescence, girls mature physically and mentally about two years ahead of boys; but then boys seem to overtake them in academic ambition and physical prowess, while most girls adopt a passive role in keeping with the expectations of society. Yet both sexes share a surging physical, emotional and mental strength, coupled with a powerful sexual drive and a growing sense of independence and individuality.

Since it is generally true that these characteristics are encouraged in boys and suppressed in girls, both sexes can feel a great sense of conflict. Girls who want to compete in a man's world may not be encouraged to do so, then may indulge

A feeling of independence will prompt many adolescents to venture out into the world to earn their own money.

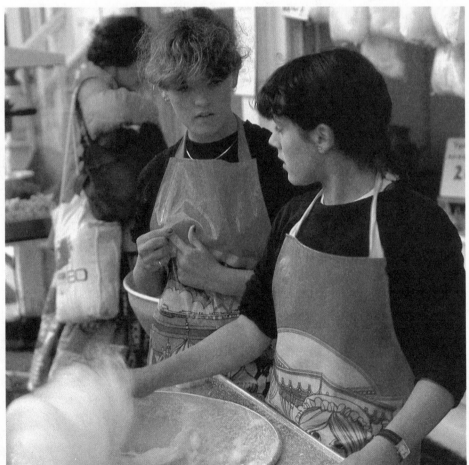

Sally and Richard Greenhill

Q Our eldest daughter was nothing but trouble all the time she was in her teens. But our second girl is as quiet as a mouse and doesn't give us a moment's worry. Is this significant?

A Not really. The amount of trouble children are in adolescence isn't necessarily an indication of how they will behave in adult life.

Parents often worry about their first child. This is mainly because they are adjusting to the responsibilities of parenthood and so the child may be under pressures which make him or her react strongly. A younger child is not under so much pressure and so is likely to behave differently. But if you think your second daughter is too quiet, you should seek advice from a professional counsellor.

Q I found a collection of dirty magazines under my son's bed. What should I do?

A Adolescents tend to be preoccupied with sex. All you need to do is to point out that they offend *you* and that you would rather he did not leave them where you can find them. If you make too much of a fuss they could take on the attraction of forbidden fruit.
But what are you doing looking under his bed in the first place? After all, they were out of sight. It sounds as though he's more considerate of you than you are of him—and is probably more able to handle 'adult' thoughts than you give him credit for.

Q My teenager has begun to ask me the most bizarre questions about God, the meaning of life, and so forth. Is this normal?

A Yes, in fact it's probably the sign of a lively, enquiring mind grappling with some of the fundamental questions of life. Adolescence is a period when growing children begin to be fascinated by obscure and often seemingly pointless questions—and impatient with adults who, having become adjusted to the existence of death, whether or not there is a God, or the state of the world, show little interest in discussing these matters. But they can be of profound interest to adolescents, who are aware of them as topics for the first time.

in rebellious behaviour; boys who display sensitivity and many of the caring traits encouraged in girls often have trouble relating to both sexes, who are brought up to expect 'masculine' behaviour in boys.

Young men have just as difficult a time in many ways as girls. Not only are they expected to be 'strong', both physically and in their support of the opposite (and supposedly weaker) sex, but they are also expected to be successful providers. This can place a great burden on the male adolescent who may be frightened of failure in both respects, and this may cause him to revert to child-like behaviour when under stress.

Contradictory and confused behaviour can worry and annoy parents, who have perhaps forgotten that they went through exactly the same turmoil. It needs great patience to cope with an individual who demands to be treated as an adult one minute and then throws a fit of temper or demands help, support and reassurance, just like a child, the next.

How can parents help?
The most important thing that parents can do to help adolescent children is to become less obviously their protectors and disciplinarians, while still remaining a 'safety net' should problems arise.

Obviously, this change has to take

place over a period of time, ending whe the children have reached a recognize state of adulthood and feel they are read to leave home and fend for themselves.

Though they are reluctant to admit i adolescents really do rely very much o their parents. This is the time of life whe they are trying to work things out fo themselves, but they still need someon to turn to for support when a situation be comes too difficult for them to cope with.

What is 'normal' behaviour?
Sometimes the various kinds of exper mentation or rebellion in which adoles cents may become involved can get out o control, yet the children will not admi anything to their parents. How can yo tell if things have got out of hand?

The mental state of adolescents is ofte very confusing to an outsider. The par ental cry most often heard by doctors is 'I'm sure he—or she—isn't normal . . .'

Moodiness, an entirely normal—bu usually temporary—stage, can result i the adoption of unconventional or out landish points of view, and these can als be very disturbing. In the main, there i no great significance in this stage mental development, although it ma seem at times morbid for a health youngster to be preoccupied with death o religion, or just pure obstinacy for

Normal behaviour in adolescence

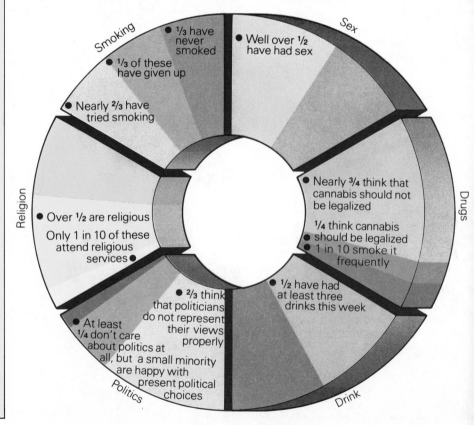

Smoking
- 1/3 have never smoked
- 1/3 of these have given up
- Nearly 2/3 have tried smoking

Sex
- Well over 1/2 have had sex

Drugs
- Nearly 3/4 think that cannabis should not be legalized
- 1/4 think cannabis should be legalized
- 1 in 10 smoke it frequently

Drink
- 1/2 have had at least three drinks this week

Politics
- 2/3 think that politicians do not represent their views properly
- At least 1/4 don't care about politics at all, but a small minority are happy with present political choices

Religion
- Over 1/2 are religious
- Only 1 in 10 of these attend religious services

eenager to hold forth noisily on left or ight-wing politics to parents who are of he opposite persuasion.

Danger signals

The most common problem in adolesence is depression. This can be either a eaction to some event—such as the ailure of an important examination, the nability to find a job, the loss of a boy or irl friend—or can simply 'come from vithin' happening for no apparent exernal reason. The symptom is always eep apathy. The young person shows no nterest in anything, is listless, uncomunicative and mopes about. Sleeping abits are disturbed, he or she may wake arly in the morning, continue to lie wake, and then stay in bed complaining f tiredness long after everyone else is up. Unfortunately, there is an increasing rend of teenage depression leading to uicide—or attempted suicide. It is vital o watch for danger signals such as deep ntrospection, furtive behaviour, drinkng or outbursts of aggression and iolence. Do not try to play amateur sychiatrist or put a label on why a child eems depressed. If there appears to be ny cause for concern or anxiety, ask for utside help. It is far better to play safe an be sorry.

Drug abuse is sometimes a worry to paents of adolescent children. However, al-

dolescents often feel out of tune with the st of society and form close friendships ith their equals.

though cannabis use among teenagers has increased over the past decade, it has not been associated with a noticeable shift in truancy nor a lowering of grades. Contrary to the 'stepping stone' theory, cannibis use is not usually followed by the use of other, 'hard', drugs.

However, evidence that an adolescent is using other drugs such as amphetamines, 'speed', heroin, morphine, 'crack' – and even glue sniffing – should be viewed with concern. Prompt medical treatment and counselling are essential.

The use of alcohol is also a potential problem for teenagers. Although experimentation with alcohol and drugs seems to be a normal part of adolescent behaviour today, it is prolonged heavy and daily use which is of concern. Parents should be aware of the effect of their own drug and alcohol consumption behaviour on their children.

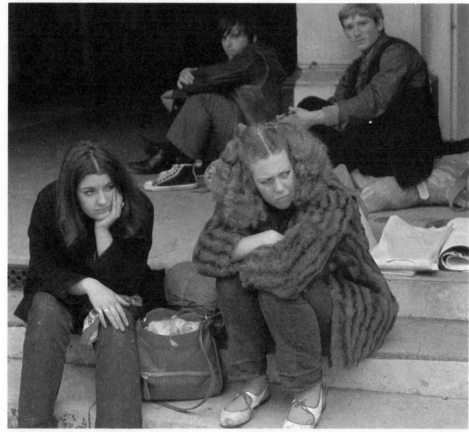

Rex Features

Sally and Richard Greenhill

Social problems

Rowdiness and vandalism cause great concern both to parents and the general public. Unfortunately, such anti-social activities can be part of growing up and proving independence. The adolescent, having rejected the security of the home but not yet ready to take on the adult world, finds security in a group of friends who have devised their own rules about dress and conduct.

Groups such as skinheads, rockers or punks are bound by strong ties within and hostility to other groups, which can, in extreme cases, erupt in gang warfare. But those who become involved in serious violence more often than not come from violent or deprived homes and so adolescence is not necessarily the root cause.

Sexual problems

To adolescents themselves, sex poses perhaps the biggest problem of all. Many are confused by their awakening sexual instincts and some may react either by becoming introspective and shy or by behaving outrageously. They need time to adjust their self-image to include this new aspect to their lives.

An important part of their development will be a growing interest in the opposite sex. Dating, going out and getting to know a number of different boyfriends or girlfriends is the way they learn to relate to people in adult life.

Part of any relationship with the opposite sex will invariably involve some sexual experimentation, as both sexes explore their own and each other's physical and emotional responses to sex.

There is, of course, no guaranteed formula that parents can adopt to ensure that teenagers do not find themselves involved in premature sexual relationships. But good sex education both at home and at school may be a way of ensuring that adolescents do understand about sex, responsibility and birth control. This means that parents and teachers need to be sympathetic, sensitive and able to discuss sexuality in a straightforward and caring manner.

Another worry for parents may be that their child will become a homosexual, especially if he or she is not interested in the opposite sex. But at this stage in life it is entirely normal for young people to enjoy close relationships with others of their own sex and this does not mean that they will be homosexual in adult life.

Setting an example

The way parents themselves behave can be crucial in dealing with adolescent problems. The example they set their children is far more important than giving them moral lectures. If they show sympathy and understanding, and make constant efforts to communicate, they will give their children the best chance of overcoming adolescent problems and becoming well-adjusted adults.

Problems which may affect adolescents

Problems	Reasons	Signs	How parents should react
Depressed behaviour	Inability to make friends; school or exam problems; loss of boyfriend/girlfriend; bad self-image; anxiety about the state of the world; no apparent reason	Apathy; introspection; secrecy; tiredness; bad schoolwork; disturbed sleep; surliness; difficulty in communicating or refusal to communicate at all; threats of suicide	Consult the school as to the situation; ask advice from family doctor or psychologist; bolster child's self-esteem in terms of appearance and ego; never shout 'Snap out of it!'; ask yourself: are you expecting too much? Are you caring enough?
Promiscuity (sleeping around)	Insecurity; anxiety; curiosity; confusion about the part sex plays in forming relationships	Staying out very late or all night; contraceptive devices hidden or obvious taking of the Pill; secrecy concerning a close relationship; rebelliousness	Try to talk about it calmly; be supportive, never react with horror; discuss responsibility and contraception; if you know you can't discuss without embarrassment find someone who can—a friend, your doctor or counsellor
Excessive slimming (affects girls more than boys)	Possible psychological rejection of female sexuality or fear of male sexuality	Bad self-image; consistent loss of weight; starvation due to dislike and refusal of food; self-induced vomiting after being persuaded to eat	Consult doctor/psychologist; be reassuring; don't panic!
Alcohol and drug abuse	Depression; parents do same; too-easy access; defiance of parents; bravado; insecurity; boredom; like the taste; like its effect; identification with drug cultural life-style; denial of, or escape from, real life	*Alcohol:* drunken behaviour *Cannabis:* cough, sore eyes, lethargy *Stimulants:* over-activity, fast, incoherent speech *Hard drugs:* needle marks in arms, scratching due to itching skin, yawning, sweating *Glue:* sores around mouth and nose, drunken behaviour	Check with school; consult doctor/psychologist/counsellor
Rowdiness and vandalism	Proving independence; rejection of home rules in favour of gang's rules; rejection of society's values; rejection of environment	Aggression; acts of violence against property and individuals	Consult psychologist/counsellor

Adrenal glands

Q My father suffers from high blood pressure when he gets excited and he is always saying it is the fault of his adrenals. Could this be true?

A Raised blood pressure is one of the symptoms of certain rare adrenal diseases, but such a disease is unlikely to be the cause of your father's problem. Other factors, among them heavy smoking, being overweight or under stress, are much more likely to be responsible for high blood pressure.

If your father is under constant pressure at work, or if he has an excitable temperament, it could be that his adrenals are continually being required to produce adrenalin—the hormone that enables us to cope in emergencies—and consequently his body is not being allowed to return to normal, so the excessive adrenalin in his system could, in time, have led to high blood pressure. But this is not the same as saying that it is the fault of the adrenals themselves.

Q I have been advised to have my adrenals removed. Is it possible to have this done and still live normally?

A Yes. Patients who must have their adrenals removed for medical reasons are able to lead a perfectly normal life by taking cortisone regularly. So you can stop worrying.

Q I have been overweight since I was a child. I have tried dieting, exercise— everything. Could there be something wrong with my adrenal glands that causes this problem?

A If your excess weight is distributed evenly all over your body, the answer must be no. There is only one disease of the adrenals which gives rise to obesity: Cushing's syndrome— and this is extremely rare. It is very easy to spot because there is an obviously uneven distribution of fat on the body: the arms and legs remain thin and fat is concentrated on the chest and abdomen. If you really want to get to the root of your obesity, the first thing you must do is to go and see your doctor.

Most people have heard of the adrenal glands, but few would claim to know where they are and what they do. They are, in fact, vital to many of the body's normal functions—and are particularly necessary to us in resisting infection and coping with stress.

The adrenal glands—known as the adrenals—are located immediately above the kidneys where they sit, like caps, one on top of each kidney. Each gland consists of two distinct parts: the inner medulla and the outer covering, called the cortex. These parts secrete different hormones, each of which has an entirely separate function.

The adrenal medulla

The medulla, or core, of the adrenals is the part of the gland which secretes adrenalin and its close relation, noradrenalin. Together these are known as the 'fight or flight' hormones because they prepare the body for the extra effort required to meet danger, cope with stress or carry out a difficult task.

The adrenal medulla is unique among those hormone-producing glands known as the endocrine glands in that it is closely connected to the nervous system. This is exactly as you would expect of the gland responsible for priming the body to be ready for instant action.

The adrenal glands, which are located just above the kidneys, have two distinct parts performing quite different functions.

Today, the dangers and stresses we face are as likely to be psychological as physical, but either way, the body has the same physical reaction. There is a surge in the production of adrenalin which makes the heart beat faster and more strongly. This raises the blood pressure, while at the same time constricting the blood vessels near the surface of the body and in the gut, re-directing the flow of blood towards the heart—the reason we go 'white with fear'. It also turns glycogen stored in the liver and muscles into glucose required for extra energy.

When the danger is over or the stress removed, adrenalin production is reduced and the body returns to normal. However,

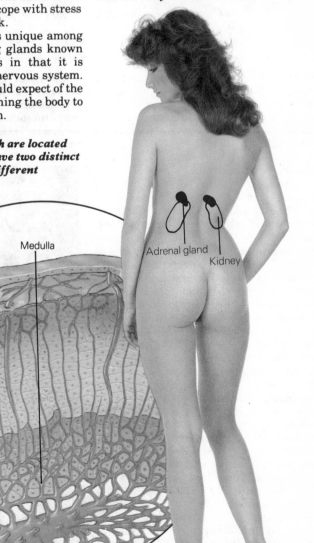

Cortex   Medulla

Adrenal gland

Kidney

Frank Kennard

Hormones and their uses

Source	Hormone	Functions	How synthetic hormones are used as drugs
Adrenal medulla	Adrenalin	Prepares body for physical action (see illustration)	To treat a heart attack In severe allergic collapse During surgery, mixed with local anaesthetic
	Noradrenalin	Maintains even blood pressure	To treat a heart attack
Adrenal cortex	Aldosterone	Regulates excretion of salt by kidney Keeps balance of salt (sodium) and potassium Plays a part in the body's use of carbohydrates	As replacement therapy
	Cortisone	Stimulates manufacture and storage of energy-giving glucose Reduces inflammation Regulates distribution of fat in the body	As replacement therapy when adrenals are missing or defective As replacement therapy when pituitary is defective In shock after severe injuries or burns In severe allergic reactions In rheumatoid arthritis (either as tablets or injected into painful joints) and related diseases In skin diseases such as eczema (as ointment) In anti-cancer treatment, especially when lymphatic system is affected To prevent rejection after transplants
	Sex hormones	Supplement sex hormones secreted by gonads	To correct deficiencies In sex-related areas (e.g. contraception) To promote muscle and bone growth

if the danger or stress is constant, or if we are continually over-excited or under pressure, the body remains primed for action – and in time this can lead to stress-related conditions (e.g. high blood pressure).

The adrenal cortex
Wrapped around the adrenal core, the adrenal cortex secretes a series of hormones known as steroids, the most important of which are aldosterone and cortisone.

Aldosterone: There are three types of steroids, each one performing a quite different function. The first, known as the 'salt and water' hormones, increase the water retention in the body. The principal hormone in this category is aldosterone, which acts as a chemical messenger and tells the kidneys to reduce the amount of salt being lost in the urine.

Salt determines the volume of blood in circulation, which in turn affects the heart's efficiency as a pump. Every molecule of salt in the body is accompanied by a large number of water molecules. This means that in losing a lot of salt, the body loses even more water, and this reduces the volume and pressure of the circulating blood. As a result, the heart has difficulty in pumping enough blood around the body.

The secretion of aldosterone is controlled by the hormone renin which is produced by the kidneys. The system

The physical signs of the effects of adrenalin can frequently be seen in professional sporting events, among both the participating players and the spectators. John McEnroe often exhibits the characteristics associated with adrenalin.

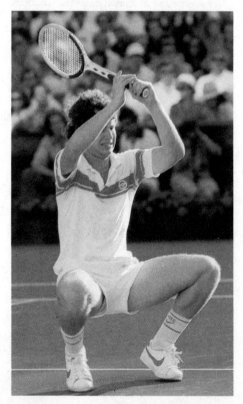

works rather like a see-saw: when aldosterone is low, the kidneys produce renin and the hormone level rises; when it is too high, the kidneys reduce their level of activity and the amount of hormone present in the blood returns to a normal level.

Cortisone: The sugar hormones, of which the most important is cortisone, are responsible for raising the level of glucose in the blood. Glucose is the body's principal fuel, and when extra amounts are needed, as in times of stress, cortisone triggers off the conversion of protein into glucose.

Many hormones act to push up the level of sugar in the blood, but cortisone is the most important. By contrast, there is only one hormone that keeps the level down, insulin. Because of this imbalance, there is more likely to be a deficiency, a condition which is known as diabetes and which is treated with insulin in the form of tablets or injections.

As well as playing a key part in metabolism (the life-maintaining processes of the body), cortisone is also vital to the functioning of the immune system, which is the body's defence against illness and injury. But if the normal level of cortisone is raised through medical treatment (for example, to prevent rejection after transplant surgery), the resistance to infection is reduced. However, the body does not produce excessive cortisone naturally.

Effects of adrenalin
(the fight or flight hormone) on the body

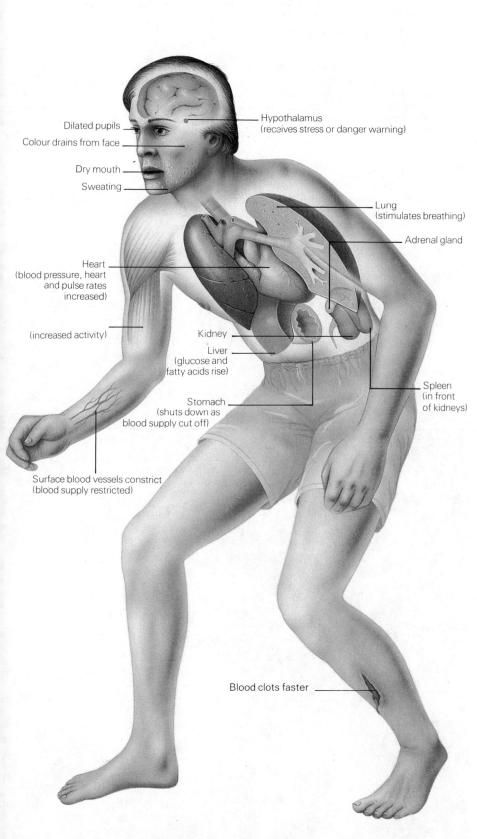

Dilated pupils

Colour drains from face

Dry mouth

Sweating

Hypothalamus
(receives stress or danger warning)

Lung
(stimulates breathing)

Adrenal gland

Heart
(blood pressure, heart
and pulse rates
increased)

(increased activity)

Kidney

Liver
(glucose and
fatty acids rise)

Stomach
(shuts down as
blood supply cut off)

Spleen
(in front
of kidneys)

Surface blood vessels constrict
(blood supply restricted)

Blood clots faster

Sex hormones: The final group of hormones produced by the adrenals are those known as the adrenal sex hormones. These are secreted by the adrenal medulla and they complement those produced in even larger quantities by the gonads, or sex glands.

The principal male sex hormone—also present in women to a lesser degree—is testosterone, which is responsible for increasing the size of muscles. Anabolic steroids are synthetic derivatives of male sex hormones.

Control of cortisone

Cortisone is so crucial to body function that its secretion needs to be under strict control. The mechanism which regulates its production – and that of steroids – is another endocrine gland, the pituitary, situated at the base of the brain.

The pituitary secretes the hormone ACTH, which stimulates cortisone production and, as with the hormones renin and aldosterone, the two substances work in a see-saw action known as a feedback mechanism. When the cortisone is too low, the pituitary secretes ACTH and the level rises; when it is too high, the gland slows production and the level of cortisone falls.

Cortisone as a drug

Cortisone is used as a replacement treatment in the debilitating hormonal disorder known as Addison's disease, of which President John F. Kennedy was a sufferer. When this condition occurs, either the adrenal cortex does not produce sufficient cortisone of its own or the pituitary gland is defective.

As a drug, it is also valuable for a number of other complaints—though it is best used as a short-term remedy. Because it reduces inflammation, it is used in the particularly painful form of arthritis called rheumatoid arthritis and related rheumatoid diseases, for skin complaints such as eczema, and in certain allergic reactions such as asthma or drug allergies.

It is also given to overcome the natural immune reaction so that the body will not reject 'foreign' tissue in transplant operations, and in combination with drugs, to treat cancers.

Steroid therapy is not without its dangers, however. The most serious drawback is that the adrenal cortex is likely to stop producing its own cortisone when synthetic cortisone or a related drug is given for any length of time.

Diseases of the adrenal glands are rare, but occasionally they do go wrong.

Nevertheless, today, with a wide range of replacement hormone treatments serious consequences can be avoided.

Ageing

Q **I am in my twenties and am already a heavy smoker. Will this affect my life expectancy?**

A Pulling no punches, the answer has to be yes. Many people underestimate the risk they are taking by smoking 25 cigarettes a day (even low tar brands). Smoking will almost invariably accelerate the ageing process, often causing death before the age of 60 from heart disease and diseases of the lungs and arteries. It is easy to lump together the dangers of car and airplane crashes, stress and obesity, and say that smoking is a minor hazard by comparison. It is not; it is a major cause of premature death.

Q **I have always had a very active and satisfactory sex life, and it worries me that I may lose interest as I grow older. Is this likely to happen?**

A Not necessarily. Libido does seem to be reduced with old age, but there is no reason for sexual activity to disappear from your life. It is thought that a decrease in sexual desire may be related to the physical changes that occur in the sexual organs with age. After the menopause the vagina is not so well lubricated and a woman may need to use a lubricating jelly to ensure that penetration is easy and painless. An older man will usually find that he is slower to become erect and ejaculate. However, there is no reason for these things to inhibit your lovemaking in later life. Many men and women enjoy sex well into their eighties.

Q **I have noticed that my mother who is well into her seventies, has definitely shrunk over the last couple of years. Is this normal?**

A Yes. The main reasons for height loss are thinning of the spinal bones and wearing down of the cartilage in between them. Old people's backs also tend to bow slightly, so that they bend forward a little. Trying to maintain a correct posture in earlier life will probably help the vertebrae and the connecting muscles to maintain their strength a little, and this could possibly help to reduce height loss in old age.

The saying 'You're as old as you feel' is more true today than it's ever been because medical advances and improved living conditions are making a healthy and happy old age a reality.

A century ago in Britain a male child who survived his first year could expect to live to be 48, a female 50. Today, many people in the developed world live well into old age. Indeed, the average life expectancy has now reached 70 for men and 76 for women.

Why we live longer
The vast improvement in our life expectancy is largely the result of public health measures. Better sanitation and an improved standard of living have eradicated many of the conditions that tend to encourage disease, and mass immunization programmes have protected children from diseases which killed in the past. New methods of treating disease, such as antibiotics, radiotherapy and transplants, also help save lives.

The increase in the number of older people has led to an expansion in the field of geriatric medicine. Its aim is to alleviate the diseases and disabilities of older people.

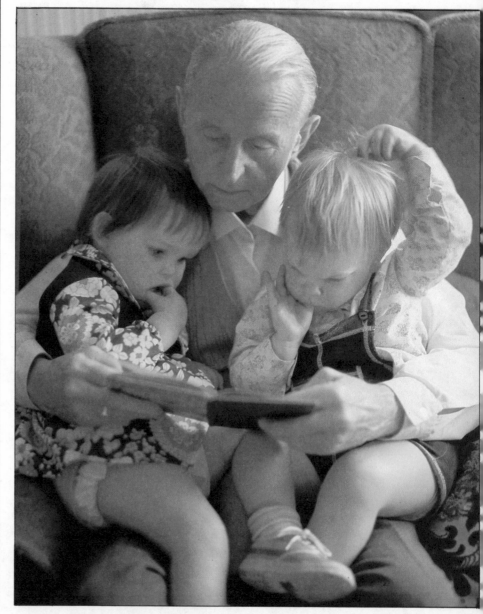

he causes of ageing

he reasons for the differences between eople in life expectancy lie in a mbination of factors, such as the genes eople inherit from their parents (that tal part of cells which determines our herited characteristics), and their other's health during pregnancy, both which can have an effect on longevity. igarette smoking and drinking to excess an undermine health, as can living in oor conditions.

Thus the peak of physical, mental, exual and social well-being varies from erson to person and may be greatly ifluenced by a whole range of elements. or example, a successful businessman ay be in his prime at 50, enjoying good ealth, but if he is made redundant his tuation may change overnight—and the sychological effects of being out of work an be far-reaching, causing him to age aster than previously.

he importance of heredity

person who comes from a long-lived amily will generally have a long life, espite any adverse conditions. And just s genetic inheritance has a part to play i determining life expectancy, so, too, it ffects the health and strength of idividual organs. A 'good' inheritance vill mean that a person is more likely to ave a strong heart, a healthy brain and harp eyesight and hearing.

Unfortunately, there is nothing anyone an do about the genes they inherit—no ne can choose their parents or go back in ime and change them. However, ndividuals who have inherited 'bad' enes might be able to live out their otential life-span to its full—and live a easonably long life—if they take care to ry and minimize any of the risk factors hat cause, or at least contribute to, ill-.ealth and ageing.

Environment

'ortunately, genetic inheritance can only xplain some of the traits that appear to un in families. Many physical and nental patterns can only be explained by he shared environment of parents and hildren. Overweight mothers are more ikely to have fat children—though this is nore than likely due to their 'inheriting' heir mother's eating habits, rather than er genes.

Similarly, bronchitics may have chesty children who grow into bronchitic adults because their parents smoked and there was enough smoke in the home environment to affect the children's lungs. It is also true that they are more likely to mitate their parents and smoke themselves, becoming more liable to lung complaints.

The facts about ageing

- Skin loses its bloom and elasticity, causing wrinkling especially around the eyes and mouth.

- Hair turns grey, then white, becoming sparse—baldness in men starts between 20 and 30, and this is a progressive condition.

- Eyesight deteriorates and eyes are more prone to cataracts.

- A loss of calcium makes bones brittle and liable to fracture. Spinal bones become thinner, resulting in height loss and stooping.

- Loss of teeth, frequently caused through gum disease, alters facial structure.

- The body's balance and gait alters with diminished height and stiffening joints, making the body's carriage less stable.

- Smoking causes heart, circulatory and lung problems.

- Alcohol can damage the liver and nervous system.

And how to stay healthy

- Avoid exposure to the sun and wind. Moisturize and handle the skin gently.

- Keep off certain drugs, like cannabis, in youth—research suggests that this could cause premature hair loss.

- A relatively straightforward operation can cure cataracts.

- Modern advances in hormone treatment can't reverse these changes, but can help to halt or, at least, slow the process down Your doctor will advise you about any risks involved.

- Have regular dental check-ups and maintain an effective oral hygiene routine.

- Take gentle exercise regularly from youth to middle age, older people should avoid strenuous sports—such exertions can cause bones to crack.

- Stop smoking.

- Drink moderately.

The risk of a short life—whether due to inherited or environmental factors—can be greatly reduced if people ensure that they lead a healthy life, especially in later years; eating the right balance of different foods, taking regular exercise, practising routine safety precautions both at home and at work and cutting out smoking can all help to increase potential life-span.

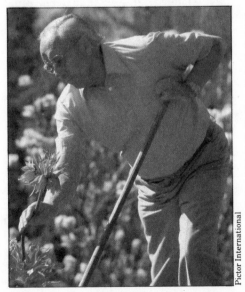

Pictor International

Cell ageing

Common health problems which may increase with age are not in fact caused by the ageing process itself—arthritis has the same causes no matter what the age of the individual. But certain conditions are more likely to occur in later years simply because of a general decline in the body's strength and resistance to infection. This happens as a result of cell ageing.

Most of the body's cells are continually renewing themselves as they wear out. Exact replicas of the old cells are made by a process of cell division, in which cells simply divide into two. The chief exception to this rule is the brain, the cells of which cease division after birth.

As the body ages, the cells begin to deteriorate and function less efficiently, some of which can be explained by general wear and tear on the body. For example, the skin can be compared to a piece of elastic which, on being stretched, will return to its original shape; gradually, with use, it loses its elasticity and remains permanently stretched.

Various theories have been put forward to explain the loss of the body's cellular efficiency. One is that some of the body's cells have a built-in life cycle. A 'programme' switches them on and off—and an example of this can be seen in

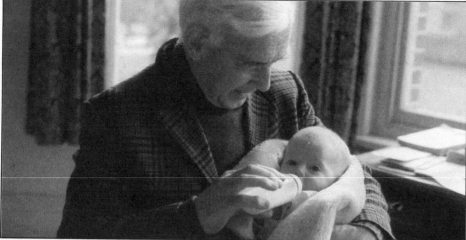

Spectrum

It is important that older people who may otherwise feel isolated experience continuing sense of involvement and have directions in which to channel the affection. A grandchild, or even a pet, can fulfil that need.

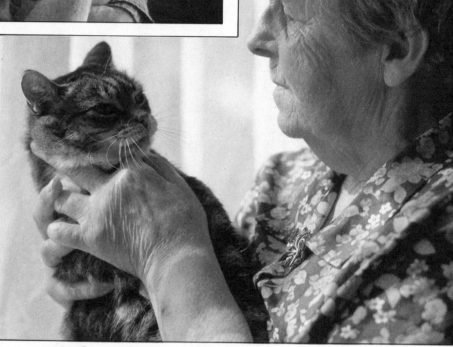

declining muscle strength. In old age certain cells do switch off, causing muscle fibres to decrease in size, but recent research suggests that this decrease can be counteracted, to some extent, by regular exercising throughout middle age and even in later life.

Another theory is called the 'Hayflick limit'. This says that our cells seem to have a predetermined number of cell divisions; once they have divided a certain number of times, they simply stop dividing. Even a small difference in the interval between cell divisions could radically alter a person's life expectancy.

A third theory states that cells gradually fail to reproduce themselves as accurately as before. This can lead to the death of the cell or the production of a whole series of cells which are not as efficient as the original.

The only explanation for the deterioration of brain cells, which are unable to reproduce themselves, is that they just fail to work as efficiently with time, or perhaps as a result of viral diseases.

There is also evidence to suggest that the body's immune system can break down in old age. Normally it produces antibodies which attack foreign cells, which may invade the body as a result of infection, but sometimes the body fails to distinguish foreign cells and it reacts by attacking some of its own cells.

Why women live longer

Women outlive men by an average of five to six years. Various explanations have been given for this, but many of them have little supporting evidence. Some people believe that women are under less stress than men because women usually do not hold such demanding or responsible positions.

Others say that this is nonsense and that quite the reverse is true: women have to deal with far more stress than men, but they learn to cope with it better.

The fact that, until recently, women have smoked far less than men, could certainly be a contributory factor to female longevity. However, younger women are smoking far more today and this could cause a radical change in their life expectancy.

It has been suggested that female hormones may play a significant part in women's longer life expectancy by protecting them in some way. But research in this area is still inconclusive. However, contrary to this view, there is evidence that the drop in the level of female sex hormones after the menopause can have the opposite effect. The lack of the hormone oestrogen can accelerate wrinkling and cause the vagina to become less well lubricated. Also, the body's calcium balance can be affected and this makes women more susceptible to osteoporosis (thinning of the bones). This condition makes bones more likely to fracture and can caus bowing of the spine. Hormone replac ment therapy can be preventive although this treatment has some risk which should be carefully considered consultation with a doctor.

Benefits of retirement

In the past, old people occupied an autho atitive and well respected role in societ This role has gradually been undermine young people being considered mor capable of dealing with newer, mor scientific methods of working, as well a being thought more creative. One of th effects of these views has been th increase in early retirement–and th can make older people feel useless an unwanted. But in fact many of them fin that it gives them the opportunity the have been waiting for to take up nev interests and hobbies. The adage 'You'r only as old as you feel' may be a cliché, bu it rings very true for many people.

AIDS

Q Where can I get more information and advice regarding AIDS?

A The US Public Health Service operates an AIDS hotline. The toll-free number is 1-800-342-AIDS. Information is also available from your local Red Cross Chapter.

Q Can someone contract AIDS from being bitten by a mosquito?

A A good deal of research centering on this as a possible route of infection has been conducted. Much of it has been carried out in Africa, where mosquitoes are well known for their ability to carry and transmit the organism that causes malaria. All the evidence indicates that people cannot be infected with the AIDS virus from the bite of any insect.

Q How are hospitals going to be able to handle all the AIDS cases predicted in the years ahead?

A That's a very good question, one for which there are no easy answers. In some major cities, entire hospitals have been converted into facilities devoted to the care and treatment of only AIDS patients. That may be helpful now, but many new hospitals and clinics will no doubt be needed in the not too distant future.

Q Can I get AIDS from *giving* blood?

A No. It is not possible to contract the disease from the procedure used to extract blood. At no time does a person donating blood ever come into contact with the blood of another person.

Q How can I tell if someone has been infected with the virus that causes AIDS?

A You can't, unless they have already developed the symptoms of the syndrome. The AIDS virus may remain dormant within a person for several months or years before producing any symptoms—if ever.

When a group of eminent scientists was asked about the prospects for finding a cure to AIDS, 19 per cent predicted its eradication by the year 2000. Even under this optimistic minority forecast, the toll in human lives will be enormous.

In 1979, doctors in both San Francisco and New York found themselves dealing with an unusual outbreak of a type of cancer that is only rarely encountered outside of Africa. The malignancy, called Kaposi's sarcoma, primarily affects the blood-vessel tissues of the skin. Up until that time, its infrequent occurence in the US usually involved older males of Italian or Jewish background. The patients in New York and San Francisco, however, were mostly young white men, and the majority were homosexual.

It was also noticed that many of these men were particularly susceptible to a variety of infections. One of these, *Pneumocystis carinii*, was caused by a one-celled organism that is normally harmless in humans. The search for explanations for the cancers and infections led to a surprising discovery: all of the patients had severely depressed immune systems. In 1981, the new disease was described and given a name: acquired immune deficiency syndrome, quickly shortened to the acronym AIDS.

When members of two other groups, intravenous drug users and individuals who had received frequent blood transfusions, were found to be suffering from the disease, suggesting that some sort of infectious agent in the blood might be responsible, the search for the possible cause of AIDS began in earnest.

The cause
It is now known that AIDS is caused by a retrovirus, designated HIV (human immuno-deficiency virus), one of a small family of viruses that reproduce in a particular way in host cells. HIV is able to invade several different kinds of cells in the body, but its affinity for certain white blood cells of the human immune system, T4 lymphocytes, is what lies behind the virus's ability to cause the syndrome. T4 cells, sometimes called helper T cells, help to regulate the activity of other components of the immune system.

Once inside a T4 cell, the AIDS virus uses an enzyme called reverse transcriptase to translate its genetic message, which is in the form of RNA (ribonucleic acid), into DNA (deoxyribonucleic acid). The viral DNA then inserts itself into the host cell's chromosomes where it may remain inactive until it is 'triggered', perhaps by a new infection, to instruct the host cell to begin rapidly making numerous copies of the virus. The T4 cell dies, probably from perforations of the cell wall by the escaping viruses.

During Gay Pride Week in New York in 1983, homosexuals took to the streets in an attempt to get the authorities to pour more money into research on AIDS. So far, no effective form of treatment exists to combat this killer disease.

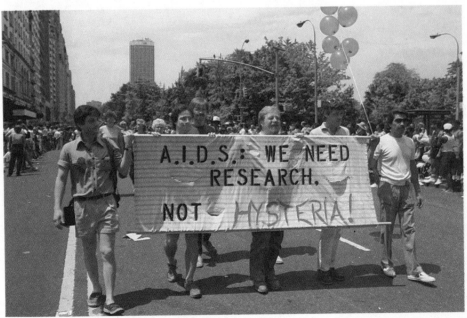

The decline in the number of helper T cells cripples the immune system and renders the body vulnerable to the many opportunistic infections that characterize AIDS.

Who is at risk?
Anyone who comes into intimate contact with the body fluids of an individual carrying the HIV virus is at risk of becoming infected and then possibly developing AIDS in the future.

As of 1987, sexually active homosexual and bisexual men accounted for over half of the recorded cases of the disease in the US. The principal means by which the AIDS virus is transmitted between members of this group is anal intercourse.

More than one-third of AIDS patients have been intravenous drug users, who acquire and pass along the HIV virus by sharing contaminated hypodermic needles with other users. The number of AIDS victims in this group as a percentage of the total is rapidly growing.

Also increasing is the percentage of cases attributed to heterosexual contact with an infected partner. It has been estimated that between 4 and 7 per cent of all adult AIDS patients contracted the disease in this way.

A pregnant woman infected with the HIV virus can give the virus to her child during the pregnancy or at the time of birth. Researchers believe the chance that a baby born to an AIDS patient will become infected is roughly 50 per cent.

Before a test for screening donated blood was developed in 1985, a very small number of transfusion recipients became infected. The chance of contracting AIDS by this route is now very remote. A relatively high percentage of hemophiliacs acquired the HIV virus through injections of clotting factors, which are derived from thousands of donors. New techniques for removing viruses from such material have greatly reduced the risk for this group.

All present evidence strongly suggests that casual contact with an infected individual in the home, workplace or school does not pose a threat.

Symptoms
A person can be infected with the HIV virus for years before suffering any symptoms or developing a full-blown case of AIDS.

The very earliest signs of infection might be swelling of lymph glands in the neck and armpit, sometimes called persistent generalized lymphadenopathy (or PGL). A later development may be a condition called AIDS-related complex (or ARC). Symptoms include fever, fatigue, loss of weight, diarrhea, and attacks of shingles or herpes.

Full-blown AIDS is characterized by the collapse of the immune system which leads to the severe opportunistic infections and cancers, such as Kaposi's sarcoma, that eventually prove fatal.

The HIV virus can also invade cells in the brain. Dementia, which is similar to Alzheimer's disease, and even schizophrenia may occur as a result either early or late in the course of the disease.

It is believed that not all infected individuals will develop the disease. Several possible explanations have been proposed. Some strains of the virus may be more virulent than others. It has also been suggested that certain co-factors—another infection or even a genetic susceptibility—might enhance or trigger the virus's ability to cause disease.

Testing
Individuals infected with the HIV virus develop antibodies against it. While this response appears to fall far short of effectively dealing with the invader, the antibodies make it possible to test the blood to detect their presence, which is a clear sign of infection.

The testing of blood supplies has, at least in the US and Europe, virtually eliminated the risk of contracting AIDS from medical transfusions.

The widespread testing of individuals has proved problematic and controversial. Furthermore, a negative test result does not necessarily guarantee that a person is AIDS-free, since the period of time between actual infection and the production of antibodies may be four weeks to four months and sometimes as long as a year.

Treatment
At present, there is no cure for AIDS. Treatment primarily involves administering antibiotics to combat infections as they occur and taking appropriate courses of action to deal with the other conditions associated with the disease.

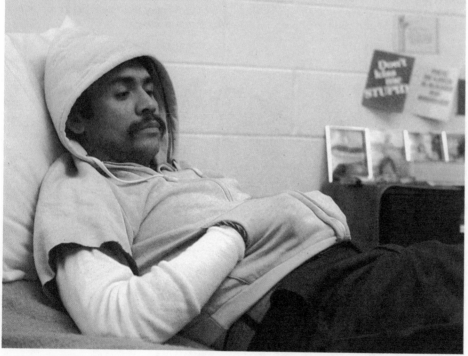

Frank Fournier/Contact Colorific!

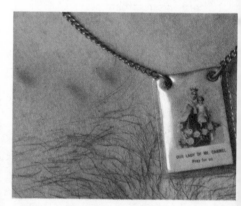

Kaposi's sarcoma (above) is a rare form of cancer, and before the emergence of AIDS, it was rarely found in young men. Homosexual men are more prone to this particular sign of AIDS.

This young AIDS victim (left) contracted the disease through the use of intravenous drugs. Drug users also run a high risk of contracting hepatitis B—both these conditions occur when dirty needles are used to inject drugs.

Many antiviral drugs have been tested against HIV in the laboratory and several have undergone limited human trials. The most promising of these is azidothymidine, or AZT, manufactured under the brand name Retrovir. While it has been shown to inhibit the ability of the virus to reproduce in some patients, the drug has proved less effective in others. It can also produce serious side effects, including suppression of bone marrow leading to severe anemia.

Prevention

Until a vaccine that provides protection against the AIDS virus is available, the only way to prevent infection is to avoid those practices that have so far been responsible for the spread of the disease.

The use of condoms among homosexuals and heterosexuals has become commonplace. Promiscuous contact with numerous sex partners is properly discouraged. And steps to reduce the use of contaminated needles among drug users, who represent the principal vector of transmission to the heterosexual community, have been either proposed or undertaken.

Most attempts to produce a vaccine that would confer immunity to the AIDS virus have made use of proteins located in the virus's outer envelope. Introduction of such material into an uninfected person should cause their immune system to produce antibodies against any future invasion of the real virus. Other potential vaccines would rely on another virus, such as the vaccinia virus used in smallpox vaccines, to deliver the HIV gene for

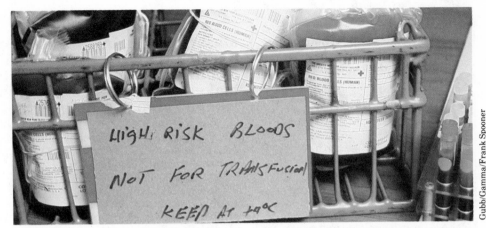

Since it was discovered that AIDS could be transmitted through blood transfusions, great efforts have been made to discourage high-risk donors.

the antibody-stimulating protein. Still other vaccines might use attenuated, or weakened, HIV to produce antibodies. Because the AIDS virus mutates easily, coming up with a vaccine effective against all potential strains may prove difficult. That any vaccine will be safe is not certain, but research in this area still continues.

The discovery of a second AIDS-causing retrovirus in West Africa, designated HIV-2, further complicates the vaccine picture. Antibodies to HIV-2 are not detectable with current screening tests and it is unlikely that an HIV-1 vaccine, if one were available, would offer any protection against the new virus.

The scope of the epidemic

The World Health Organization estimates that as many as 10 million individuals worldwide may already carry the AIDS virus, and that a tenfold increase in that figure within five years is a real possibility. The US Public Health Service puts the number of people infected in the US at close to 1.5 million, and suggests that five years from now approximately one-quarter of them will have AIDS. Barring a breakthrough in treatment or prevention, according to one estimate the death toll in the US could reach 179,000 by the end of 1991.

With no effective cure as yet available, it is particularly important that AIDS patients are given careful counselling and emotional support, for example in self-help groups, to help them come to terms with their condition.

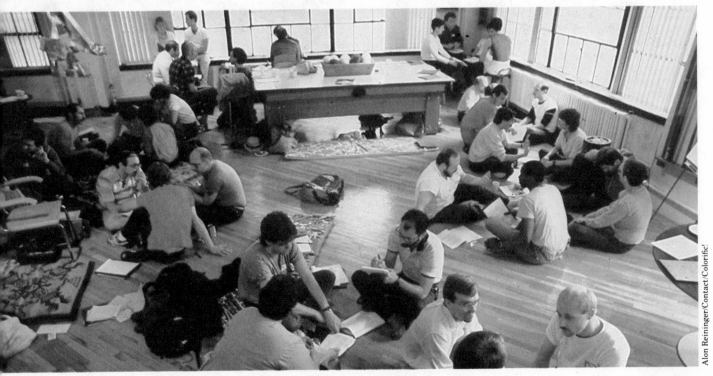

Alcoholism

Q I have heard that women are more at risk when they drink than men. Is there any truth in this?

A Drinking among women is on the increase. Not only is it now accepted that they can go into bars on their own, but they can also buy alcohol from the supermarket. Generally speaking, however, women still drink less than men—and so they come to less harm. But if a woman becomes an alcoholic she is more vulnerable to the effects than a man; her liver is likely to be affected earlier than a man's, and treatment is often not as satisfactory. Then there is the problem of the alcoholic expectant mother—she risks causing mental retardation in her baby, and it may also be born with congenital deformities such as dislocation of the hips or a cleft palate.

Q My brother-in-law drinks an awful lot, and in the last year I have noticed a marked change in his personality. He used to be pleasant and outgoing—now he is surly and introverted. Could his drinking be the cause of this?

A Almost certainly. Very heavy drinkers can become moody, violent and jealous, or think they are being persecuted. Even worse, they can have trouble in remembering things, they may hear imaginary voices, see visions and become unable to cope with life. All this can result in *delirium tremens,* the symptoms of which are trembling, sweating and a feeling of panic. If you recognize any of these danger signs in your brother-in-law, he should be encouraged to seek help as soon as possible.

Q Where can I go to get help for alcoholism?

A Go to your doctor for advice on physical aspects of alcohol addiction—he or she will refer you to a clinic if necessary. For family problems—and any others you may have—see a social worker. There are also self-help groups such as Alcoholics Anonymous, which can provide long-term help and support for anyone who wants to kick the habit.

Most people drink moderately, enjoy it, and come to no harm. But there are those who become so dependent on alcohol that they are unable to lead a normal life. This makes it vital to recognize the danger signals and to know when to stop.

When people talk about alcohol, they are usually referring to drinks which contain varying amounts of pure alcohol. Alcoholic drinks have a restricted food value in the form of sugar (as in sweet wines, for example) and carbohydrate (in liquor and beers made from grain), but basically alcohol is a drug—that is, a substance which affects the workings of the mind and body in a variety of different ways.

Taken in moderation, alcohol can encourage the appetite and produce a feeling of well-being. This is because the alcohol stimulates the blood flow to the skin which has the effect of making the drinker feel pleasantly warm. When it reaches the brain anxiety is reduced and self-confidence increases. Shyness seems to disappear, and the world becomes a happier, more affable place.

Dependency

Heavy drinking, however, is quite another matter. If it is repeated over an period of time, subtle changes can occur in the personality—it is thought that these have a chemical basis—and this can lead to the need to carry on the drinking pattern. When this feeling becomes so persistent that every time a drink is delayed there is an urgent desire to have another, a state known as 'dependency' has been reached.

In the early stages of heavy drinking this dependency tends to be psychological rather than physical. After all, it is anxiety and stress that usually lead people into drinking in the first place, but then they come to rely on the alcohol as a prop to keep them at their ease.

Unfortunately, if the drinking becomes

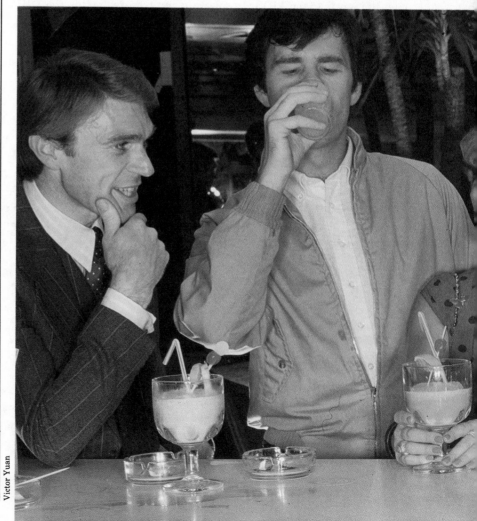

Victor Yuan

much heavier, so does the psychological need. In the transitional period this may not be noticeable, but as physical dependence grows, withdrawal will become more and more difficult and uncomfortable. Eventually, deprivation for any length of time will result in the trembling, sweating and acute stress. The first drink will always relieve these feelings—until the next time, and there is always a 'next time'.

Alcohol and personality changes

Alcohol tends to affect different people in different ways. The same amount can turn one person into the 'life and soul' of the party, bring out violent aggression in another, and merely send a third quietly to sleep.

Although it reduces tension, alcohol is not a stimulant, but a depressant. As soon as it enters the bloodstream, it begins to impair judgement, self-control and skill. Research has shown that workers with blood alcohol levels of between 0.03% (30mg, or the equivalent of two cans of 6.4 beer) and 0.1% (100mg) have considerably more accidents than those with less than 30mg.

With driving, the likelihood of having an accident increases when the blood alcohol level reaches 30mg; at 80mg, it is four times greater; and at 150mg it is 25 times greater. This is because the co-ordination between hand and eye and the ability to judge distances deteriorates progressively.

The problems of alcoholism

Once an excessive drinker is unable to stop drinking without outside help, he or she can be classified as an alcoholic. And it is in this situation that the social, economic and medical problems—often already self-evident in the heavy drinker—can worsen, bringing despair and confusion to the life of the alcoholic—and everyone else with whom he or she has contact.

Alcohol breaks up marriages, sets children against parents, and vice-versa, and costs individuals their jobs and their reputation in the community. Ultimately, of course, it can also kill.

When most people think of alcoholics, they visualize 'winos', 'bums' and down-and-out inebriates, but it is not just the deprived and inadequate members of our society who resort to the bottle as a means of escape—there are children too inebriated to take in their school lessons after lunch, businessmen incapable of working in the afternoons, and housewives barely able to prepare a meal at the end of the day.

Alcoholism can strike irrespective of age, class, creed, color or sex, and once afflicted, alcoholics will mix only with like-minded friends, neglect their families, break promises, lie and steal, and live only to drink.

Reasons for heavy drinking

Drinking is an accepted and approved cultural activity. As such, it would appear that some people are more exposed to the risk of becoming alcoholics than others simply because of social pressures and conditioning. For example,

Drinking with friends is a relaxing way to unwind. But drinking for its own sake or showing a marked reluctance to stop, no matter how much has been drunk, are danger signals. Any one of these people (below) is potentially a 'problem' drinker, not just the 'obvious' one.

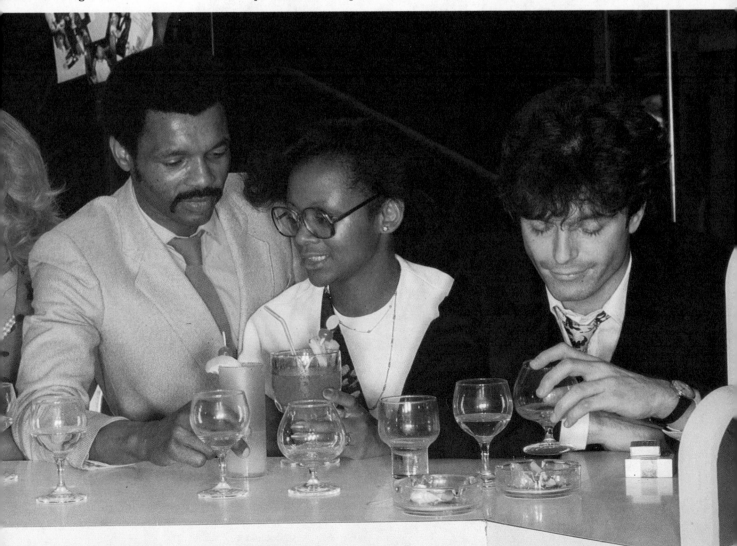

Q What is the best cure for a hangover? I get a terrible headache and everyone has different ideas on what I should do about it.

A The only real cure for a hangover is rest. Phencticin may be used to treat a bad headache, but aspirin should be left well alone. It will only cause further disturbance to an already irritated stomach. The 'hair of the dog' remedy (having another drink) is not recommended: it will simply lead to spending the rest of the day in bed in a drunken haze. As you say, everyone has their own pet cure—orange juice, vitamin pills, egg milkshake, but the rule to follow is that prevention is better than cure. Drink as much water as possible before going to sleep after a drinking session. Dehydration is the main cause of a hangover and water will help reduce this effect of alcohol. But (to pursue the subject to its obvious conclusion) it is still best to try not to drink too much and to avoid having hangovers altogether.

Q Are some people more vulnerable to alcohol than others? I seem to get drunk on one glass of wine.

A It used to be thought that people who found themselves in trouble over drinking were different in their physical and psychological make-up to others, but this is now thought to be untrue. Anyone can become an alcoholic and if you find you do not respond too well to alcohol, try to avoid it. If everyone knew their limits and stuck to them firmly, the problem of alcoholism with all its risks would be greatly reduced.

Q My sister says her husband has a drinking problem, but denies that he is an alcoholic. Is this possible?

A No. They are one and the same thing. Someone whose drinking over a period of time has made him dependent on drink and who may do harm to himself and others is an alcoholic—though he and his family may not wish to see the real nature of the condition. But sooner or later—and the sooner the better—they are going to have to face it for what it is.

The effects of alcoholism

Physical

- Cirrhosis of the liver—there is no cure for this most common disease associated with alcoholism

- Other diseases—alcoholics commonly develop kidney trouble, heart disease and ulcers, which fail to respond to normal treatment

- Frequent appearance of bruises and cuts resulting from falls and bumping into things

- Persistent vague physical complaints with no apparent cause, like headaches and stomach upsets

- Coarse inexplicable trembling of the hands; sweating

- Loss of appetite and insomnia

- Pins and needles in hands and feet

- Delirium tremens—sometimes accompanied by frightening hallucinations

Emotional and social

- Alcoholics suffer increasingly from anxiety, depression, remorse and phobic fears

- Obsession with drink overrides all else of importance in life and the need for drink increases as tolerance grows

- Disruption or breakdown of family life and persistent marital problems

- Loss of friends and interests—alcoholics seek the company of others like themselves

- Frequent absenteeism from work and repeated job changes, with a loss of efficiency and reliability that can lead to job loss

- Lack of concentration and loss of memory

- Behaviour and social adjustment lower than previously experienced

- Shabby appearance, poor hygiene

- Surreptitious drinking, gulping of drinks

- Arrests for drunken driving

studies of national groups reveal that the Irish have a high rate of alcoholism; in contrast, the Jews' rate is very low. Certain professions seem to encourage alcoholism—traveling salesmen, bar-people and company directors, among others, are particularly at risk. Presumably, extensive socializing and the availability of drink are responsible in these cases.

The housewife is increasingly a victim of this form of addiction. Often isolated, either with small children or with too little to do once a family has grown up and left home, drinking can provide her with a welcome escape from an apparently humdrum existence. And the fact that most supermarkets today stock alcohol makes it only too easy for her to buy it as part of her routine shopping.

In most cases, drinking starts at an early age, with children, not surrisingly, copying the habits of their parents. It is statistically proven that the children of alcoholic parents have a higher than average risk of developing the problem themselves. Teenagers also tend to be strongly influenced by their friends' behavior, and the largest population of problem drinkers in the country is among single urban males under 25.

Today, so much socializing is built around the consumption of alcohol that it is hard to avoid it. You may easily find yourself mixing with others who drink, going to the same place regularly for this purpose, becoming accustomed to the lights, sounds and smells. In adddition, advertising suggests that men are not men unless they drink, and drunkenness is a sign of masculinity. Finally, a refusal to drink is usually considered to be abnormal and often seen as a deliberately anti-social action. All these factors can combine to make it difficult to maintain a responsible attitude to alcohol.

Danger signals

The body develops a tolerance to alcohol, and the danger lies in the fact that more drinks are soon needed to reproduce the original feeling of relaxation and well-being. The higher the daily intake becomes, the more difficult it is to give it up. If an individual drinks to relieve worries, this can lead to an escalation in drinking: more worries mean more alcohol, and fewer worries become the reason for a round of celebratory drinks.

It can take between 10 and 15 years for someone to develop an addiction to the point where they can be classified as an alcoholic. But symptoms to watch for are an obvious obsession with alcohol and the inability to give it up or even restrict drinking to a reasonable level, moral and physical deterioration, and obvious work, money and family problems. The typical alcoholic will probably need a drink early in the morning and may need continual boosters to keep going during the day.

Safe drinking

In a situation where an individual wants to drink, but not to excess, alcohol should be consumed as slowly as possible and some food should always be eaten beforehand so that the alcohol will be absorbed more slowly into the bloodstream. Consumption can also be kept down by interspersing alcoholic drinks with non-alcoholic ones. It is better not to drink alone, as it is all too easy to consume more than usual just in order to combat feelings of loneliness.

If you do not want to drink, you should not feel shy about saying so. And if you know how much you can drink before going over the top, simply set a limit to the number of drinks you accept and stick to it.

Finally, the combination of drinking and driving—or handling any type of machinery—is extremely dangerous. In fact, 16 percent of individuals involved in accidents at work, 22 percent of those in home accidents and 30 percent of those in highway accidents have elevated blood alcohol levels.

People who know they will be drinking should leave the car at home or take a non-drinker along to drive. Or they should leave the car behind and take a taxi or get a ride. There should not be any halfway measures; the rule is clear and simple: *never drink and drive.*

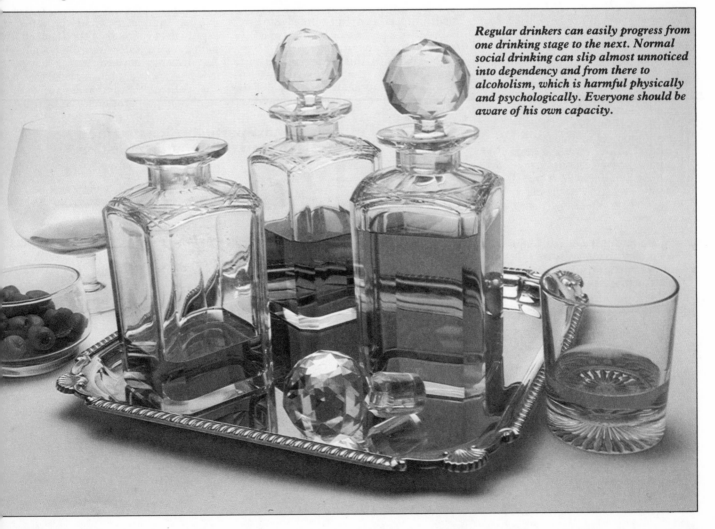

Regular drinkers can easily progress from one drinking stage to the next. Normal social drinking can slip almost unnoticed into dependency and from there to alcoholism, which is harmful physically and psychologically. Everyone should be aware of his own capacity.

Alimentary canal

The alimentary canal is where our food is digested. We are mainly unaware of this important process—so what exactly happens?

Food is the fuel that powers the activities of the body. But before it can be of any use, it must be properly processed. The body's food processing plant is the alimentary canal, a muscular tube about 10m (33 ft) long which starts at the mouth and ends at the anus, from which undigested wastes are expelled in the form of feces.

Eating

When food is put in the mouth at the beginning of its journey through the alimentary canal, it is tested for taste and temperature by the tongue. Solid food is bitten off by the front teeth (incisors), then chewed by the back teeth or molars. Even before the food is tasted, and during chewing, saliva pours into the mouth from salivary glands near the lower jaw.

Saliva moistens food, and the enzymes it contains start digestion. By the time it is ready to be swallowed, the original mouthful has been transformed into a soft ball, called a bolus, and warmed or cooled to the right temperature.

Though quick, this stage is in fact quite complex. First the tongue pushes the bolus of food up against the roof of the mouth and into the muscle-lined cavity at the back of the mouth: the pharynx.

Once food is in the pharynx, several activities take place within the space of a couple of seconds to prevent swallowing from interfering with breathing. The soft palate, the non-bony part of the roof of the mouth, is pushed upwards by the tongue to shut off the inner entrance to the nose, the vocal cords are quickly drawn together, and a flap of tissue called the epiglottis snaps down over the entrance to the tubes that lead to the lungs.

From the pharynx the bolus now passes into the oesophagus, or gullet, the tube joining the mouth to the stomach. The bolus does not just fall down the oesophagus because of gravity but is pushed along by waves of muscle action called peristalsis.

Except during eating, the oesophagus is kept closed just above where it enters the stomach by a ring of muscle called the cardiac sphincter which prevents the highly acid contents of the stomach from being regurgitated into the oesophagus. As a bolus of food passes down the oesophagus, the sphincter relaxes to open the pathway into the stomach, which relaxes in preparation for being filled.

Peristalsis—how partially digested food (chyme) is moved through the intestine

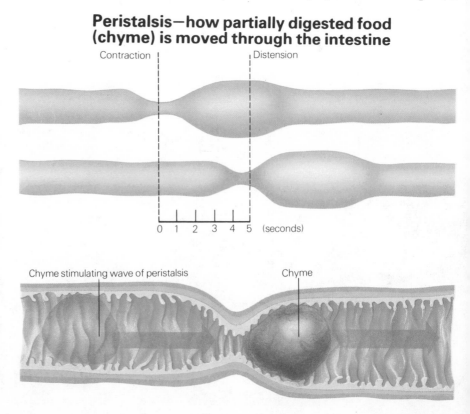

Contraction — Distension

0 1 2 3 4 5 (seconds)

Chyme stimulating wave of peristalsis

Chyme

Alimentary canal

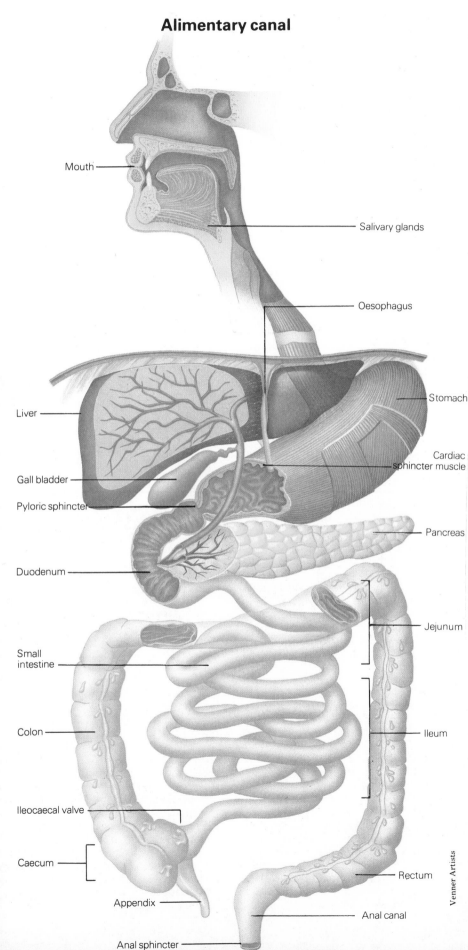

Mouth

Salivary glands

Oesophagus

Liver

Stomach

Gall bladder

Cardiac sphincter muscle

Pyloric sphincter

Pancreas

Duodenum

Small intestine

Jejunum

Colon

Ileum

Ileocaecal valve

Caecum

Rectum

Appendix

Anal canal

Anal sphincter

Venner Artists

Digestion

The stomach is a collapsible muscular bag designed to store food (so that it is not usually necessary to eat small meals all day long), to mix food with various digestive juices, then to release it slowly into the intestine.

Food is mixed as the stomach wall contracts and relaxes and is moved along by waves of peristalsis. By the time it has spent two to six hours being processed in the stomach, the partially digested food has been converted by various chemicals to a liquid called chyme.

The stomach exit is guarded by a muscle known as the pyloric sphincter, very like the sphincter at the stomach entrance, except that it is never completely closed. As the waves of peristalsis push chyme through the stomach, the

Aids to digestion

The alimentary canal processes approximately 35 tons of food during the course of an average life of 70 years. No wonder, then, that it sometimes goes wrong. Some ills of the alimentary canal are so common they have become household words—ulcers, appendicitis, constipation, diarrhoea and heartburn, to name a few. While some are unavoidable, there are ways to keep the digestive system healthy.

● Do not eat (or feed children) too much. This puts a strain on the digestion and can create a weight problem. In infants it can lead to vomiting and regurgitation.

● Chew your food properly before swallowing. The digestion of carbohydrates starts in the mouth with ptyalin, an enzyme in saliva.

● Include sufficient roughage in your diet—fruit with the skin on, lightly cooked vegetables, bran with your breakfast cereal. Dietary fibre cannot be digested by the alimentary canal but stimulates the passage of food through the large intestine, helping to prevent constipation and perhaps some intestinal diseases as well. Fibre-rich foods are useful for slimming because they are filling, but not fattening.

● Drink sparingly with meals because liquids of any kind dilute digestive juices.

● Avoid any foods you know you or your family react to badly.

● Minimize stress. This increases the acid secretion of the stomach and the muscular action of the whole system, causing food to be pushed along too fast so that it is not properly digested.

● Stop smoking, or cut down, because, like stress, it stimulates acid secretion.

Common problems in babies and children

Symptom	Related symptoms	Possible causes	Action
Diarrhoea **Babies**	Fever, appetite loss, vomiting	Infection of canal or middle ear, tonsillitis, common cold	Boiled water only, call doctor if symptoms persist more than 24 hours
		Food allergy	Boiled water only. Re-introduce foods one by one to find cause. See doctor it if persists
Diarrhoea **Children**	Fever, appetite loss, vomiting, abdominal pain	Infection of canal	Fluids for 24 hours. See doctor if symptoms persist
		Effects of antibiotic drug	Bland diet; fluids. See doctor if symptoms persist
Vomiting **Babies**	Diarrhoea, appetite loss	Too much air taken in with feed	Nipple with smaller hole. Small, frequent feeds
	Constipation	Bowel obstruction	See doctor at once
Projectile vomiting **Babies under two months**	Constipation, no appetite loss	Pyloric stenosis (see questions)	See doctor at once
Vomiting **Children**	Diarrhoea, appetite loss, abdominal pain	Appendicitis	See doctor at once
Constipation **Babies**	Vomiting	Bowel obstruction	See doctor at once
		Anxiety about potty training	Stop training temporarily
Constipation **Children**	Poor appetite	Lack of fluids, lack of exercise, too little roughage	Plenty of fluids; increase roughage

How long food is in the body

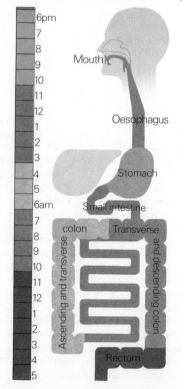

sphincter lets out chyme in small amounts into the small intestine.

The small intestine is in fact the longest section of the alimentary canal, measuring 20ft (6m) and getting its name not from its length but its width—about 1½in (4cm). The first 10in (25cm) of the small intestine is known as the duodenum, the next 8ft (2.5cm) as the jejunum and the final 11ft (3.3m) as the ileum.

The largest part of the digestive process takes place in the small intestine, through the action of digestive juices made not only by the intestine itself, but by the liver and the pancreas which are closely linked to the alimentary canal. The liver produces bile, a substance stored by the gall bladder and needed to digest fats, and the pancreas produces pancreatic secretions, which, like bile, pass into the duodenum.

As waves of peristalsis move chyme along the small intestine, it is given another thorough mixing. In the ileum, digested foodstuffs are absorbed into the blood via thousands of tiny corrugations in the gut wall called villi and carried first to the liver, then to all body cells. At the end of the ileum a sphincter called the ileocaecal valve keeps chyme trapped in the small intestine until another meal is eaten. When more food enters the stomach, the valve opens and chyme passes into the large intestine, a tube about 3ft (1.5m) long and an average 7.5 cm (3 in) in diameter.

Excretion

Anatomists divide the large intestine into four parts: the caecum, colon, rectum and anal canal. The caecum, and the worm-like appendix that extends from it, are both blind alleys with no known functions in man. In the colon, by far the largest section at 1.3 m (4½ ft), water is absorbed into the blood from the liquid remains of digestion. By the time these remains reach the rectum, they are in the form of solid feces. Rather than the continuous contractions of peristalsis, the progressively more solid remains are moved along by giant propulsions that take place only a few times a day.

Finally, feces enter the anal canal, which is kept closed by the last sphincter in the alimentary canal. In infancy the sphincter opens automatically when the anal canal is full. But as the nervous system matures, we learn to override the automatic signals.

Venner Artists

Allergies

Q I have been suffering from a food allergy for years and sometimes it really gets on top of me. What I want to know is can there be a lasting cure?

A There are several ways of relieving the symptoms of allergies, but they are not cures. Whatever treatment you receive, it is not going to change your basic sensitivity to the particular food in question.

Q My daughter's best friend has just developed an allergy to penicillin, and has terrified my daughter by claiming that she will die at the onset of the first disease she catches, as she won't be able to take penicillin to fight the infection. Surely there must be some alternative drugs to pencillin?

A There is really no need to worry. Although a penicillin allergy does reduce the number of antibiotics which a doctor might consider prescribing, there is still a range of antibiotics available for those people with this type of allergy.

Q My son of four is allergic to cats and touching them brings him out in a nasty rash. Will he grow out of this problem or will it remain with him for life?

A Possibly. Children who suffer from either allergic rashes or eczema often do grow out of those problems though they may suffer from other forms of allergy (asthma for example) when they are older because they have a basic tendency to be allergic.

Q I suffer terribly from hay fever and, as I am now pregnant, I am anxious to know whether my child could possibly inherit this condition from me?

A Unfortunately, this could happen, although it is by no means a certainty. Research shows that children of allergic parents are more likely to suffer from an allergy than other children. But there are still not enough facts available for us to fully understand why this should be so.

Allergy-sufferers sometimes have to bear considerable discomfort and inconvenience, but although there are at present no cures for allergies, medical research is making encouraging progress in discovering the many causes and alleviating the symptoms

An allergy is a sensitivity to a substance which does not normally cause people any discomfort or harm. Hay fever, which is caused by a sensitivity to pollen, is a well-known example. Asthma, eczema, rashes and a variety of other complaints can be caused partly or entirely by an allergy. In fact, allergies can affect almost any part of the body and be caused by a vast range of natural and artificial substances.

Allergies are a common complaint. Distressing though the symptoms are, quite a lot can be done to improve the situation. Running eyes and sneezing are typical of hay fever.

They are seldom life-threatening, though they can be dangerous, and are often very uncomfortable for the sufferer. They are also a great puzzle to medical science, because although many allergic conditions can be relieved by medical treatment, we still have very little idea of their basic cause.

Allergies are a reaction to allergens, a name given to those substances (such as

Di Lewis

pollen) that spark off symptoms of an allergy in someone who is sensitive to it. Among the commonest allergens are foods (notably eggs, milk and fish), pollens, spores, insect bites (especially bee and wasp stings), animal fluff (such as cat's hair) and chemicals. One type of allergy is caused by contact with metals, which explains why some people get a nasty rash from wearing certain pieces of jewellery.

A common allergen in the home is the dust mite, a tiny creature, invisible to the naked eye, which lives in bedclothes, carpets and curtains. Some people are allergic to heat or cold so that their hands swell when plunged, for example, into hot or cold water.

Symptoms

As a general rule, the symptoms of an allergy tend to show up in those parts of the body which are exposed to the allergen. So an airborne allergen, like pollen, makes its severest impact in the eyes, nose and air passages. Food allergies reveal themselves through swollen lips, stomach upsets or diarrhoea.

An allergy to a metal would affect the skin, and an allergy to rubber would result in a rash on part of your body where, for example, the elastic of your underwear came into contact with your skin. But this is only a general rule, because if an allergen gets into the bloodstream it can cause reactions almost anywhere.

This is particularly true of food allergens, which are absorbed through the digestive tract into the blood. Because of this, food allergens can cause a wide range of reactions in sufferers, including eczema, nettlerash, asthma and even mental disorders.

Skin allergies: There are really three basic forms of allergic reaction affecting the skin. The most common, particularly among children, is eczema and this appears as a rash or as scaly skin, to be found mostly on the hands, face, neck and the creases of the forearms and behind the knees.

Contact dermatitis, often caused by metal jewellery or by chemicals in washing powders, is a blistery, itchy inflammation of skin which has come into direct contact with the allergen.

There is also urticaria, best described by its popular name, hives. This is a red, irritating swelling which often has a small white point in the middle which makes it look like a nettle sting.

Eye and ear allergies: Allergic reactions can also affect the eye, and these generally show up as irritation and redness in the white of the eye. Severe

swellings can occur, but generally the symptoms are watering and soreness.

The ears, too, are sometimes the target of allergens; when this happens fluid will build up inside the ear and may temporarily affect your hearing.

Hayfever can affect the eyes and ears, though its principal target is the nose, which becomes stuffy, runny or sneezy. Unlike a common cold, which should clear up after four or five days in an

How allergy-producing histamine is released

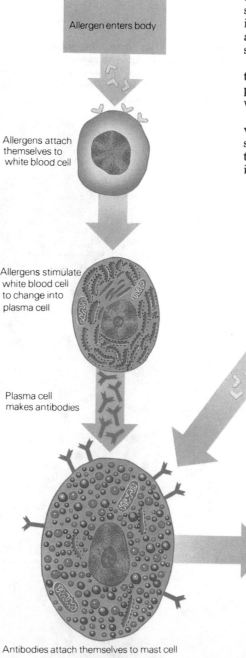

Allergen enters body

Allergens attach themselves to white blood cell

Allergens stimulate white blood cell to change into plasma cell

Plasma cell makes antibodies

Antibodies attach themselves to mast cell

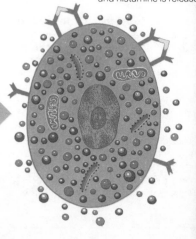

Allergens enter body for second time

Allergens and antibodies combine and histamine is released

otherwise healthy person, hayfever w last for as long as you are exposed to t particular pollen to which you a allergic.

Food allergies: These have a w variety of symptoms. The most obvio symptoms of an acute food allergy are stomach upset followed quickly nausea, vomiting or diarrhoea. Peo who are acutely sensitive to a food m also get a swollen tongue and li Sometimes the sufferer gets two kinds symptoms; for instance, a child who allergic to cow's milk may get diarrho and a skin rash. Apart from skin rash which may appear hours or even a f days after eating the food, th symptoms become apparent alm immediately after eating, usually with an hour. This makes it quite easy for t sufferer to identify the allergen.

Asthma attacks can also be brought through an allergic reaction to foods a pollen, and this is characterized wheezing, and difficulty in breathing.

Doctors now believe, however, that variety of other physical and men symptoms can be caused by food allerg though the cause can be difficult identify. Depression, anxiety, headach

Common allergies

Allergy	Allergen	Symptoms	Treatment	Prevention
Asthma	Dust mites Animal hair Pollen Some foods and food additives	Difficulty in breathing; wheezing	Prick test for diagnosis. Bronchodilator if breathing problem severe. Course of injections	Keep house dust-free. Avoid pollen; keep clear of allergic foods
Contact dermatitis	Contact with allergen, e.g. jewellery, chemicals in washing powder	Itchy, blistery inflammation	Steroid creams given on doctor's prescription	Avoid contact with allergen
Eczema	Some foods, especially cow's milk, flour, eggs; possibly some seafoods	Rash on hands face, neck, arms and legs; looks like scaly skin	Antihistamine tablets and creams given for skin condition	Take diet precautions to avoid allergen
Food allergy	Could be caused by almost any food—more commonly milk, flour, eggs; also strawberries, shellfish, nuts; some food additives	Upset stomach and general nausea; acute reaction produces swollen tongue and lips, as well as diarrhoea. If food is absorbed into bloodstream, it can produce skin rashes like eczema	Prick test. Elimination test. Provocation test for diagnosis of the allergen	Keep to diet; avoid allergenic foods
Hay fever	Pollen; may react to just one pollen or to several different types	Sore, itchy eyes, runny or stuffy nose, prolonged sneezing	Prick test to confirm allergy. Course of injections and antihistamine tablets to relieve symptoms	Course of injections before season begins. Listen to pollen count on weather report. Avoid open air. Wear dark glasses
Migraine	Usually caused by cheese, red wine, yeast extract, but not only caused by an allergy	Blinding headache	Elimination diet test if complaint due to food allergy	Avoid allergen foods
Hives	Foods Handling certain plants Hot and cold water	Red, irritating swelling with with small white point in centre	Skin condition treated with with antihistamine cream, if necessary	Avoid the allergens

izophrenia, hyperactivity in children d even convulsions have been ributed to food allergies. There have so been cases of bedwetting and cystitis ich have been blamed on food ergies.

Migraine can also be caused by certain ds. Like yoghurt, chocolate, cheese, at extracts, yeast extracts and some ds of red wine which contain a ostance called tyramine. Most people's dies can deal with tyramine, which is t an allergen or poison in itself, but ne migraine sufferers appear to lack a al enzyme which breaks tyramine wn. So when they eat these foods, ramine builds up in their blood and sets a chain of chemical events in the body ich eventually results in the migraine adache.

Another complaint which is not strictly eaking an allergy but which is caused food intolerance is coeliac disease. is is a disorder of the digestive system d its symptoms are wind and pain in the stomach after eating. Soft, smelly feces (which are full of undigested fat) and weight loss, results from the sufferer's inability to absorb food properly. Coeliac disease is basically an intolerance of gluten, one of the proteins which are found in wheat. Sufferers therefore have to avoid foods which contain this substance.

The most severe – 'though fortunately, quite rare' – symptom caused by allergy is anaphylaxis. In this instance, the patient's air passages swell and close and the blood pressure falls abruptly. This is an acute and life-threatening condition. though it can be reversed very quickly by an injection of adrenalin.

Causes

The basic difference between people who suffer from allergies and those who do not is still not known. Allergies do tend to run in families, and this may be due to an inherited characteristic in the cells which make up the immune system, which is the body's defence system against disease. But this is theory rather than proven fact.

However, it is known that most allergies are the result of an error in the immune system. The body's defence forces react to the allergen as if it were a dangerous infectious organism.

White blood cells called lymphocytes are one of the most important elements of the immune system. These cells are constantly on the look-out for foreign substances such as bacteria, viruses and proteins which are different from the body's own proteins and which may present a threat. When these white blood cells come across a potentially dangerous foreign protein they form a substance called antibody, which combines with the foreign protein and neutralizes it.

A slightly different antibody is created to deal with each foreign protein, but once it has been formed the body is able to produce it again to deal with any future 'attack' by that protein. This explains

Q **I am worried that I may become addicted to the drugs I am using to treat an allergy. Could this happen?**

A No. Nor do these drugs lose their effect if you have to keep taking them. However, they may have side-effects (antihistamines, for instance, can make you drowsy) and, like all drugs, should be treated with respect and caution.

Q **Whenever my father is near my mother her eyes run and she can't stop sneezing. Can you be allergic to people, places or animals?**

A No, you can't be allergic to a person, but there have been cases of wives who were allergic to their husbands' sperm. Some people who are acutely allergic to fish can get swollen lips from kissing someone who has just been eating fish. Allergy to animals is common, though it is the fine pieces of hair or fluff from the animal or bird which are to blame. You can only be allergic to a place if your are allergic to something found in that place—e.g. pollen.

Q **I sit next to a girl in the office who has eczema and sometimes the rash is really bad. I can't help wondering if it is infectious.**

A The simple answer is that allergies are not infectious. You cannot catch an allergy from another person, nor can you pick up a symptom—in this case eczema—of that allergy.

Q **My husband and I have both suffered badly over the years from food allergies. Our two children have shown no signs of developing allergies, but we wonder whether they can be prevented.**

A Some specialists say there is little that can be done, while others believe that some allergies can be prevented. The risk of becoming allergic to milk, for instance, may be reduced by breast-feeding rather than weaning on to cow's milk at an early age. Some specialists believe that you can reduce the risk of other food allergies by eating a more varied diet.

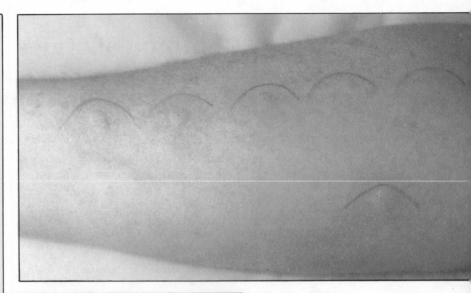

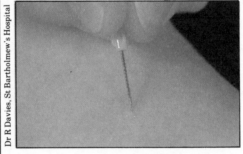

Dr R Davies, St Bartholmew's Hospital

In the prick test, the skin of the arm is pricked several times and a drop of solution (see left) containing a possible allergen is dropped on to test for a reaction. This allergy sufferer (see above) has undergone the process and found that the cause of her allergy is the dust mite. The positive reaction to this allergen is shown in the large weal at the bottom. The marks above it show no reaction and represent negative result

why we usually get infectious diseases like measles only once in our lives: after the first attack the body has supplies of antibody which can deal with the virus whenever it appears again.

By some highly complicated process, which is not yet understood by scientists, the immune system of a normal, healthy person knows how to tell the difference between a dangerous foreign protein (like a virus) and a harmless one, such as a food protein. But in an allergic person the immune system reacts to a harmless foreign protein as if it were a dangerous one, and starts forming an antibody. This antibody attaches itself to cells called mast cells. Mast cells contain a number of chemicals the most important of which is histamine.

When the body is exposed to the protein again, the antibody attached to the mast cells combines with the foreign proteins and tries to neutralize them. But in so doing it upsets the structure of the mast cell, which falls apart and releases its load of histamine. The surge of histamine produces an effect very much like the inflammation which follows a wound: it makes tiny blood vessels dilate, and as they dilate their walls become leaky, so that fluid from the blood escapes into the surrounding tissues. The dilation of the tiny blood vessels causes redness and itching, and the escaping fluid makes the

surrounding tissues swell. In hay fever the mucous glands in the nose and sinuses are also stimulated to produce fluid, which causes stuffiness and runny nose.

Diagnosis

The diagnosis of pollen allergies (and sometimes of food allergies, too) is performed with the help of a technique called the prick test. The doctor or nurse gently pricks your arm with a needle then drops a watery solution on the pricked spot. This solution contains a very small amount of one particular allergen.

Up to 40 of these little prick tests may be performed at one session without much discomfort for an adult. If you are allergic to one of the allergens, a round, red weal will show up on the spot within about fifteen minutes.

A special diet called the elimination diet is sometimes used to identify which food or foods are the cause of a food allergy. If you get better after being on this diet for several days, it is likely that one or more of the foods which have been eliminated will be the cause of your problems. You may then be asked to eat these foods again to see if your symptoms return. This process of elimination is how the identity of the allergenic food is discovered.

As elimination diets can take a long time, some doctors now use provocation tests, in which a weak solution of various foods is either injected under your skin or dropped under your tongue to see if it will provoke symptoms. As well as testing for food allergies, the doctor may also test your reaction to chemicals which are commonly found in the home or used as flavouring, colouring or preservatives in food.

Treatment

If you have the acute kind of allergy which makes you sick whenever you eat say, strawberries or shellfish, you hardly need a doctor to diagnose your complaint. The cause and the effect are obvious, and the simplest way to deal with the allergy is to avoid the allergen.

Having discovered which pollen you are allergic to, the doctor may then prescribe a course of injections. These injections also contain small amounts of the allergen, and their aim is to desensitize you by encouraging your immune system to produce a harmless 'blocking antibody'. This kind of antibody intercepts the allergen before it sets off symptoms by alighting on the mast cell antibodies.

Courses of injections can be given during the pollen season, but this method is less reliable than giving the injections before the pollen season begins. These injections do not work for everybody, but they can give about 70 per cent of sufferers protection which lasts right through the summer.

Several kinds of drug are prescribed to deal with the symptoms of allergy. Antihistamines combat the inflammatory effects of histamine when it is released. They come as tablets, liquid medicine, nose drops or eye drops, and there are injectable antihistamines which can be used to deal with serious attacks. These drugs, however, do tend to make you feel drowsy.

Another drug, disodium cromoglycate, works at the beginning of the process by preventing the mast cells from exploding. It therefore has to be taken before the symptoms occur; it can do nothing about histamine once it has been released. This drug can be given in the form of an inhalant (for asthma), eye drops (for allergic symptoms in the eye), tablets (for stomach allergies) or via another device called the insufflator, which lets you sniff it up your nose.

Corticosteroid drugs like cortisone, which are very powerful and anti-inflammatory, are sometimes prescribed for skin allergies or, via an inhaler, to combat asthma. Asthma can also be controlled by a group of drugs known as bronchodilators, so called because they dilate (open up) the bronchi (the air passages around the lungs).

It should be stressed that these drugs are not cures; they simply relieve the symptoms. Nor are they without problems. Corticosteroids have to be used sparingly and not for prolonged periods, and it is even possible to develop an allergy to antihistamines! It is important to let your doctor know if you are experiencing unpleasant side-effects from a medicine. There are many brands of anti-allergic drugs, and the doctor should be able to prescribe one which suits you better.

Food allergies can sometimes be relieved by drugs, but some doctors prefer to recommend diets which ensure that you eliminate all foods to which you have an allergic reaction.

Self-help

There is quite a lot that sufferers can do to help themselves. Obviously, if you suffer from a food or chemical allergy you should make every effort to avoid your allergens. This means that you should read the labels on food packets carefully to see whether the product contains even small amounts of the substance causing your particular allergy.

Hay fever sufferers should be careful about going out in the open air during the pollen season, especially in mid-afternoon when the pollen count is highest. Dark glasses can protect your eyes against pollen or spores, and it might be worth thinking about buying a small air conditioner for your home or car which can extract pollen from the air. Some cars now have filters in their ventilation systems which are designed to catch pollen before it enters the car.

If you are going on holiday in the late spring or early summer, bear in mind that there is usually much less pollen in the seaside air than in the middle of the countryside.

Dust mites are difficult to eliminate altogether from the home, but regular vacuum cleaning of carpets and curtains and washing of bedcovers will reduce their number. Artificial fibres in pillows and duvets are less likely to harbour dust mites than feathers.

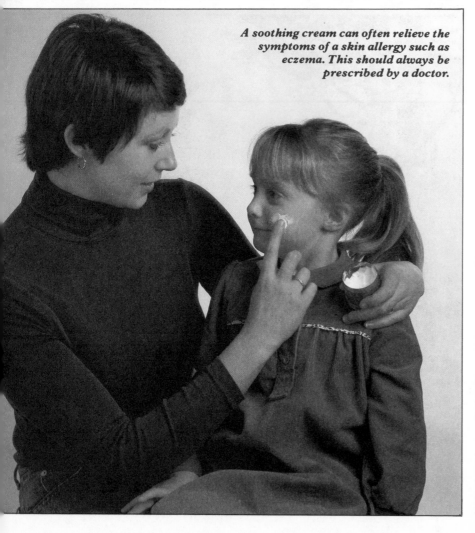

A soothing cream can often relieve the symptoms of a skin allergy such as eczema. This should always be prescribed by a doctor.

Alzheimer's disease

Q How common is Alzheimer's disease among people under 65? Is there any lower age limit?

A It is not common below age 65, and virtually unknown below the age of 45.

Q I am 47, and I keep forgetting where I put things like my car keys and my watch. I'm physically very healthy . . . but could I have Alzheimer's disease?

A It's very unlikely. All of us get absent-minded at times, especially if we are rushed or under stress. If you stay calm and take things slowly, that should solve the problem.

Q My 71-year-old mother is becoming confused, and our family doctor says she has Alzheimer's disease. I am the only child, and unmarried, and I support both my mother and myself financially. How can I get help to look after her at home? Or would care in an institution be better?

A If you live in Britain, the problem of home help can be solved by your local health authority. In the U.S., however, such help is not as readily available. Consult your physician. Depending on your means, he may recommend a private nursing service, or he might refer you to your local welfare agency. If your mother is completely helpless, and unaware of her surroundings, institutionalization is probably best.

Q I dread the thought of Alzheimer's disease when I am older. Is there any way of preventing it?

A Not at the present time. Although it is thought that raising the level of choline in the brain might help, no satisfactory method of doing this by dietary means has been discovered yet. It is, however, being explored intensively in research centres with the hope that a chemical food additive will help prevent the problem occurring.

First described by the neurologist, Alois Alzheimer, in 1906, Alzheimer's disease is a debilitating condition of the brain that usually affects people over sixty. Caused by a failure of the brain's transmission process, the symptoms include forgetfulness and loss of short-term memory.

Alzheimer's disease is a progressive, relentless deterioration of the brain that usually affects people over 60 years of age. Its onset is insidious, usually beginning with forgetfulness and loss of memory, particularly for recent events. The victim may be able to recall vividly events from childhood or early adult life, but be quite unable to remember what they had for breakfast or where they left their purse only a few minutes before.

As the disease progresses confusion may become so crippling that the patient wanders about in a daze and cannot be left alone safely, requiring constant supervision. Ultimately, total mental and physical incapacitation ensue and institutionalization is required.

The disease was first described by German neurologist, Alois Alzheimer, i 1906. Initially the term was reserved fo the occurrence of the condition in peop under 60, a synonym for it being pre senile dementia. But as autopsy studi progressed it was found that the change in demented elderly people are essentially the same as in the younge patients and it is now felt that the tw processes are different manifestations the same disease.

Most couples over sixty live a happy and relaxed life of retirement. But those who suffer from Alzheimer's disease will need increasing care and attention as the condition progresses.

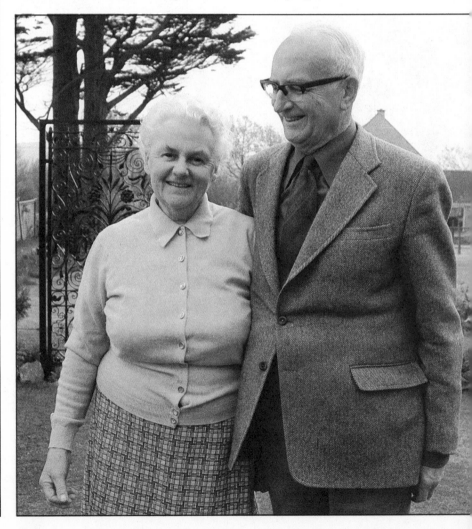

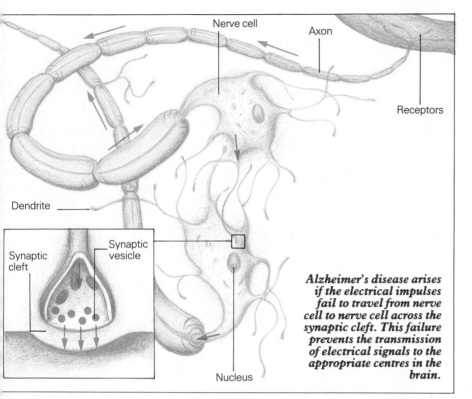

Nerve cell

Axon

Receptors

Dendrite

Synaptic cleft

Synaptic vesicle

Nucleus

Alzheimer's disease arises if the electrical impulses fail to travel from nerve cell to nerve cell across the synaptic cleft. This failure prevents the transmission of electrical signals to the appropriate centres in the brain.

When the electrical impulse reaches the synapse, it provokes the release of chemicals called neurotransmitters which cross the gap and attach to receptors on the neighbouring neuron. There the chemical message is converted back to an electric current and transmission continues. In Alzheimer's disease there appears to be a deficiency of at least one major neurotransmitter, acetylcholine or ACH, but what damages the cells to prevent their secreting the substance is not known. Moreover other neurotransmitters may be affected too.

The underlying cause remains a mystery at present but genetic factors, viral infection or even toxic damage due to aluminium or some other poison are all under investigation and show some indication of being involved in the disease. Auto immune mechanisms may also play a part.

Treatment

The deficiency of acetylcholine has led some investigators to feed large amounts of lecithen to the victims in an attempt to raise the level of choline in the blood and then in the brain. No definitive studies showing a beneficial effect have been published.

At present supportive and custodial care are the only measures available. This may impose a terrible burden on families who are responsible for elderly demented relatives. As the population shifts towards larger numbers of people over 65, this could prove to be a crisis in health care unless a cure is found.

Diagnosis

The diagnosis is largely one of exclusion since there are other diseases, such as high blood pressure, diabetes or alcoholism, which cause dementia. Some medications also cause mental confusion. After a history is obtained, various blood tests may be done to rule out these causes. An EEG (electro encephalogram) may be done to discover if there is a circumscribed area of damage in the brain due to a stroke or tumour. A newer technique, Computerized Axial Tomography or CAT scan, can demonstrate the diffuse atrophy of the brain which results from the disease. These are not specific for the diagnosis of Alzheimer's disease, however.

The finding of two distinctive lesions in the brain at postmortem examination provides the definitive diagnosis. One is the 'plaque' which is a group of dead brain cells, and the other, the 'neurofibrillary tangle' which is a twisted bundle of protein threads within the cell. These are seen in small numbers in all senile brains but are enormously increased in Alzheimer's disease.

Cause

Alzheimer's disease is due to a failure of transmission within the brain. The functioning cell within the brain is the neuron. This has a cell body which sends out short branching twigs (dendrites) on one side and a long tail (the axon) ending in similar twigs (terminal branches) on the other. Within this cell messages are

transmitted by electrical impulses from the dendrites down the axon to the terminal branches. These branches do not, however, touch the dendrites of the neighbouring neuron, being separated by a space. This entire complex is called a synapse.

This scan of a section of the brain shows the enlarged dark area typical of the presence of the disease.

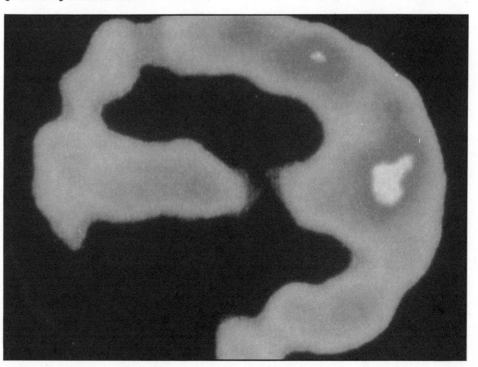

Amniocentesis

Q **Is it too late for me to start a baby? I am 39 and this is my first marriage and we would so like a child.**

A There is a good chance that you would have a healthy baby—and perhaps more than one—but don't fool yourself that there are no dangers. The risks of having a Down's syndrome child increases with the prospective mother's age, but luckily this condition can now be detected at an early stage of pregnancy. Do see your doctor and discuss the matter with him. He will refer you to a genetic counsellor if either of your medical histories show that this is a necessary precaution to ensure that you have all the information you need about any risks before becoming pregnant.

Q **Do I have a choice about whether or not to have an abortion if amniocentesis shows that my baby is going to be abnormal?**

A The decision is always left to the parents. You must imagine the life a handicapped child would have before deliberately bringing one into the world; and you should consider what would happen when you were no longer around to care for it. If you have strong objections to abortion on either moral or religious grounds, however, the final choice is obviously going to be even more difficult for you and you should discuss it with a professional counsellor or priest.

Q **I'm so terrified that having a needle stuck into my tummy will hurt. But even more important, will it hurt my baby?**

A You can be reassured on both counts. Before the needle is inserted into your abdomen, you will be given a local anaesthetic and will feel only a small pin-prick. Any discomfort is far more likely to arise from your reaction to this than from amniocentesis itself. As far as your baby is concerned, the whole purpose is to avoid injury. The needle is aimed carefully into the amniotic fluid and the ultrasound scanner will ensure that its insertion will be 100 per cent accurate

All mothers want their babies to be perfect, but until recently some mothers could not feel sure about this before the birth. Now, with amniocentesis, medical scien can help resolve these fears.

A diagnostic technique developed only in recent years, amniocentesis is used to check for abnormalities in unborn babies who may be at special risk. The test involves taking a sample of the amniotic fluid which surrounds the baby by inserting a hollow needle through the expectant mother's abdomen.

The amount of fluid withdrawn is only about 20cc, although this can vary according to the the number of tests necessary. This fluid contains cells from the fetus (the developing baby). Chemical and microscopic examinations of these can provide invaluable information, revealing the presence or absence of genetic disorders.

From about the 16th week, the doubts and fears which previously had to be endured throughout the pregnancy can be resolved. By this stage, there is enough amniotic fluid to allow the test to be carried out – and there is still time for the pregnancy to be terminated if this is thought to be necessary.

The moment the human egg is fertilized, it has all the inherited information needed to create a new being. Both male and female cells contain chromosomes, which determine sex and carry the genes that transmit inherited characteristics, but occasionally these chromosomes are found to be faulty.

What it shows

The main disorders which amniocentesis can reveal are spina bifida, an abnormality of the nervous system where the baby either does not survive or is born with severe spinal defects, and Down's syndrome. Examining the chromosomes can also reveal the sex of the baby. The sex of the baby only becomes medically important where there is known to be a history of a disorder such as haemophilia (excessive bleeding from the smallest wound) within a family. Although carried by females, the disease only affects males, and if the test reveals a male child a further test can confirm whether or not the baby is affected.

Amniocentesis is carried out quite simply, with no risk to the mother-to-be but a slight possibility of risk to the baby. A very small number of babies abort after amniocentesis and, although many would have died or aborted anyway due to abnormalities, it still means that a few normal babies are lost.

Fortunately, the technique of ultr sound scanning is now used together wi amniocentesis to give a picture of t position of the fetus in the uterus as t needle is inserted, making the procedu much safer for the unborn baby.

While amniocentesis is vital in ear pregnancy for detecting abnormalities, also serves another very useful purpo late in pregnancy in that it can reve valuable information about the develo ment of the baby.

Pregnant woman at 16 weeks

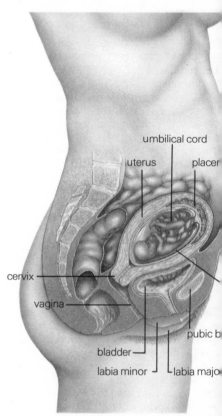

umbilical cord

uterus

placer

cervix

vagina

pubic b

bladder

labia minor

labia majo

The sample of fluid from the amniotic s is not taken until the pregnancy is advanced 16 weeks at the very earliest. This is because before then there is not enough fluid in the amniotic sac to allo a large enough sample to be taken for analysis. Also there is still time, if the parents wish it, to terminate the pregnancy if abnormalities are found.

Amphetamines

Amphetamines are powerful, habit-forming stimulants which should not be taken unless medically prescribed. What, then, are the uses and abuses of these drugs?

Q Can you become addicted to slimming pills? My aunt tried some once—but they made her depressed and in the end she got fatter than ever.

A She may have taken an amphetamine-type drug to try to suppress her appetite. But these can only be given for short periods as they can have unpleasant after-effects. Nowadays, doctors agree that the best way to lose weight is to eat less. There are now safer substitutes that can be taken instead of amphetamines—if this is really necessary.

Q I'm keen on cycle racing. Can I take amphetamines before a race to improve my staying power?

A It is not safe to do so. In fact, it is on record that a professional cyclist taking part in the Tour de France race actually died from this. As a result, all national and international sports agencies ban the use of stimulants.

Q Our little boy seems to need less sleep than we do. He's still jumping around at two in the morning. Can we give him some pills to calm him down so that we can get some sleep?

A Absolutely not. Get some professional advice at once. Your doctor will advise you whether your child is really hyperactive or just needs very little sleep. You should never give a child pills without medical advice. Remember that a dose that has been prescribed for you will be much too strong for a child—it will do more harm than good.

Q I've missed money from my handbag and I suspect my 14-year-old daughter is taking it to buy drugs. Should I confront her about the matter?

A If you feel unable to speak to her about her problems, try and get her to talk to someone she trusts. Don't accuse her of stealing until you are quite sure of the facts. She may be suffering from adolescent depression and need all the help she can get.

When first discovered in the 1930s, amphetamine was hailed as a new 'wonder drug' because its stimulant effects bring such immediate and dramatic benefits: it increases mental alertness and physical stamina, relieves depression and acts as a slimming aid by suppressing appetite. But it was soon evident that its longer term effects were anything but beneficial, particularly because it was found to be habit-forming. Prolonged use requires larger doses and can result in serious psychological and physical conditions. Consequently, its medical uses are now strictly limited and it is now rarely given.

Pure amphetamine is a colourless liquid chemical from which several stimulant drugs are manufactured,

An over-active child is difficult for parents to cope with. It was found that medically supervised use of amphetamines was effective in such cases.

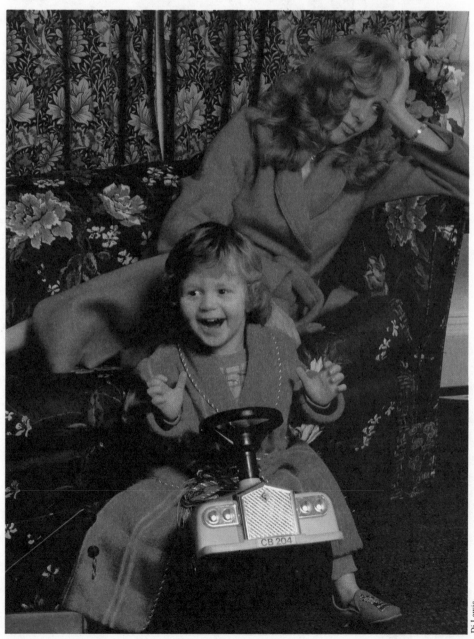

Di Lewis

Bernard Fallom Information from DHSS Prescription Statistics for Great Britain

Declining use of amphetamines

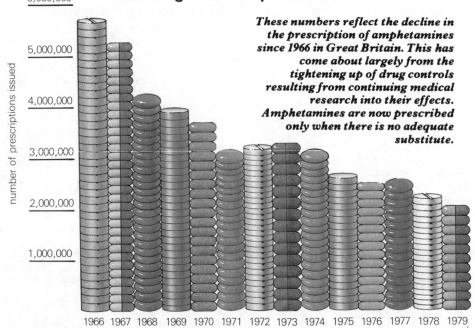

number of prescriptions issued

6,000,000
5,000,000
4,000,000
3,000,000
2,000,000
1,000,000

1966 1967 1968 1969 1970 1971 1972 1973 1974 1975 1976 1977 1978 1979

These numbers reflect the decline in the prescription of amphetamines since 1966 in Great Britain. This has come about largely from the tightening up of drug controls resulting from continuing medical research into their effects. Amphetamines are now prescribed only when there is no adequate substitute.

usually in the form of tablets or capsules. Most commonly known are amphetamine sulphate (formerly sold as Benzedrine), the stronger dextroamphetamine (Dexedrine) and methamphetamine (previously marketed as Methadrine).

How it works
Amphetamine is chemically related to the body's own stimulant, adrenalin, and this enables it to mimic many of its effects. Adrenalin is released in the body in response to fear, excitement and physical activity. Both amphetamine and adrenalin prepare the body for what has been called 'fight or flight'.

The main action of amphetamine is to stimulate certain areas of the brain, so producing increased mental alertness, greater physical movement and more rapid breathing.

Even intelligence appears to improve—in fact, an average increase of eight points has been measured on the IQ scale. Through its influence on the nervous system, amphetamine produces other physical signs, like widening of the pupils of the eyes, and affects the normal movements of the intestine, stomach and bladder; the appetite also tends to be suppressed.

Medical uses
Amphetamine was first used in the treatment of an unusual condition known as narcolepsy, where the patient is constantly dropping off to sleep. This is still an accepted use today. In addition, it has been given for depression, Parkinsonism, epilepsy, and as a tonic and to

counteract the depressant effects of barbiturate drugs and alcohol.

It has also been prescribed for bed-wetting and over-active children, because, paradoxically, it has been found to have a calming effect. However, it is important to remember that stimulants should never be given to children for this purpose unless prescribed by a doctor, and then only in the recommended dosage. This rule, of course, also applies to adult users who should know never to take drugs except on a doctor's order.

Slimming dangerously
In the 1950s, amphetamines were thought to cause little harm when taken as 'pep pills' and were also widely prescribed for women who had trouble in losing weight. Experience eventually proved that amphetamine-type drugs can only assist temporarily in the slimming process—none of the other effects are thought to be significant in helping weight-loss. Unfortunately, by the time the risks had been recognized, there were already thousands of patients dependent on them. It took some time for legal controls to be tightened.

The body does not become physically dependent on the drug, as it does with alcohol or barbiturates, but, nevertheless, there can be serious psychological hazards if it is withdrawn suddenly. This 'let-down' effect shows itself in extreme fatigue, lengthy sleep and increased appetite. Another consequence of prolonged use which can be serious is listlessness and depression.

It has therefore become accepted that

amphetamines should be used only for short periods in the treatment of obesity, taken in moderate doses and always combined with other measures, such as a low calorie diet. Some doctors take a stronger line and prefer not to use them at all for this purpose. There are now a great number of effective alternative appetite-suppressants in use which you can obtain on your doctor's prescription.

Drug abuse
In the 1960s, a new jargon and culture developed around the illegal use of amphetamines by youngsters who were often inadequate and insecure in other ways. 'Purple hearts' (which were indeed, heart-shaped until the manufacturers changed their shape), 'bennies' and 'black bombers' were among the names given to those taken by mouth. 'Speed' was the name given to injected amphetamines and the user was known as a 'speed freak'. Obtaining them often involved theft or illegal manufacture and sale. This uncontrolled use had serious consequences for many young people whose health and lives suffered greatly as a result. This affected not only them but their families and friends as well. In some cases the harm was long-term because of the disruption it caused at an important time of intellectual and emotional growth in their lives.

The risks of dependency
Those who become dependent on amphetamines are prone to accidents; they become aggressive and violent. They may have mental breakdowns, which result in delusions and hallucinations. Chronic amphetamine dependency can cause symptoms very similar to schizophrenia—an acute personality disorder often requiring hospitalization.

If an overdose has been taken, the signs in the victim are talkativeness, restlessness and trembling. Other signs are headache, flushing, irregular heartbeat, excessive sweating and stomach disturbances. In extreme cases, convulsions, unconsciousness and bleeding in the brain may occur.

To treat an overdose, the patient is given a sedative and a substance such as ammonium chloride which hastens the excretion of the drug in the urine.

Unfortunately, withdrawal cannot take place all at once, but must be carried out in gradual steps under professional supervision.

Perhaps the message that the uncontrolled use of amphetamines can be very dangerous is finally getting through. Certainly, their illegal use is declining and, hopefully, this will continue.

Amyotrophic lateral sclerosis

Q Can this condition be confused with senility or multiple sclerosis?

A It certainly cannot be confused with senility, but there are similarities with multiple sclerosis. Important points of difference are that in multiple sclerosis the patients tend to lose bladder control and there is often loss of sensation of the skin. This never happens in amyotrophic lateral sclerosis and it is very rare for sufferers to be incontinent.

Q Is amyotrophic lateral sclerosis painful?

A No. On rare occasions, however, the patient may suffer considerable discomfort with night cramp. It is well to remember that while night cramp is a very common symptom, amyotrophic lateral sclerosis is an extremely rare problem, so suffering night cramp by no means indicates that you have amyotrophic lateral sclerosis.

Q Is amyotrophic lateral sclerosis infectious? If someone in the family has the disease can it spread to others?

A No. There is no evidence at all to suggest that the disease is in any way infectious. A similar condition reached epidemic proportions in the pacific island of Guam during the Second World War, but this was recognised to be the result of an inherited abnormality running in families rather than the spread of infection. Although doctors are suspicious that the disease may be caused by a virus, no virus has yet been isolated in sufferers.

Q Can this condition run in the family?

A The cause of the vast majority of cases that develop later in life is unknown. However, there are one or two very rare diseases with similar symptoms which are known to run in families. In some cases diseases such as this have been blamed on the inheritance of an abnormal gene.

Doctors do not know the cause of this rare wasting disease which paralyzes the nerves and muscles. But it is not a painful or infectious condition.

Nerves from the brain responsible for moving muscles are called motor neurons. They have only two components to transmit the electrical message rapidly: the upper portion, known as the upper motor neuron, runs from a cell station in the brain called a Betz cell, down the spinal cord to a level where it leaves as a spinal nerve supply to particular muscles. Here there is a second cell station from which a lower motor neuron takes over and runs out to the muscles which move limbs. Amyotrophic lateral sclerosis, also known as Lou Gehrig's disease, is incurable, as these cell stations and neurons waste away.

Symptoms and treatment
No one really knows but the theory is that infection with a virus may be at the root of the problem. The main symptom is paralysis. While paralysis affects the nerves supplying the limbs and the lower trunk the patient loses only movement. But when the paralysis spreads—as it normally does—to involve the muscles of breathing and swallowing, patients have to be treated with mechanical ventilators for a short time. It is very unusual to see the condition in people aged below 25-30: the incidence rises from then on, reaching a peak around 50-60. Men are much more commonly affected than women are. Although patients can live with it for several years, the condition is fatal. The signs that develop depend very much on the extent of the disease: in the lower motor neuron it results in the typical wasting of the muscle; in the upper motor neuron the limbs grow weak and stiff and reflexes increase. The disease often affects speech and swallowing.

Physiotherapy gives the patient enormous moral support but there is no effective treatment for the disease itself.

The path of the motor neuron

Amyotrophic lateral sclerosis can arise as a result of wasting in either the upper or lower neurons. The symptoms may differ.

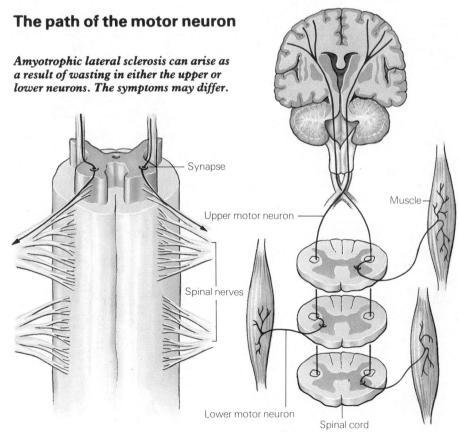

Synapse

Upper motor neuron

Muscle

Spinal nerves

Lower motor neuron

Spinal cord

Frank Kennard

Anaemia

Q I am pregnant and seem to be getting paler and paler. Could I be anaemic?

A During pregnancy the body's demands for various essential nutrients, such as iron and folic acid, are increased. The developing fetus depletes the mother's natural store by absorbing them via the placenta, and this means the mother may become deficient. This can result in anaemia, unless extra supplies of iron and folate are given. Check with your doctor and, if you do prove to be anaemic, he will give you a prescription for the pills you need to help you.

Q Can stress and strain cause anaemia? I have a very demanding job and seem to be continually tired.

A Anaemia cannot be caused by emotional problems alone; there is always an 'organic' basis. However, chronic depression, for instance, may be acompanied by a poor diet and this may eventually lead to anaemia through vitamin and iron deficiency. Have a chat with your doctor. You may simply be in need of a break.

Q I have heard that it is possible to prevent anaemia by the use of various tonics. Is this true?

A No. A normal diet, including meat, milk, fresh fruit and vegetables, will provide all the chemicals required to make blood. There is no benefit to be gained from tonics or vitamins bought over the counter.

Q My mother suffers from anaemia. I am worried that I or my children might have inherited it. Is this possible?

A Well, it depends on the type of anaemia in question. Some rare anemias such as Thalassaemia are passed on from generation to generation. In cases like pernicious anaemia the disease is not transmitted, but other family members are more likely to be affected. Common anaemias, like iron deficiency do not have a heritable basis.

People who look pale and feel run down often assume they are anaemic, but this is not necessarily so. And even if the condition is diagnosed, treatment is usually simple, quick and effective, giving a rapid return of health and energy.

Anaemia is the name given to a disorder of the blood, the composition of which is defective in some way. It is the red blood cells that are affected. These are produced in the bone marrow, and contain an essential ingredient, haemoglobin. This substance has the remarkable ability to carry oxygen, which it picks up in the lungs and then distributes to the tissues of the body where it is needed to provide energy.

The marrow produces two million red cells a second and these survive in the bloodstream for about 120 days. If the level of blood cells in circulation is reduced from normal levels for any reason, this results in a lack of oxygen reaching the tissues and produces the classic symptoms of anaemia: a lack of energy, fainting, and skin pallor.

Causes

In general, anaemia is a superfici symptom of something else that is wro in the body, and because of this there a a number of causes, the most common which is a lack of iron. Iron is a miner which is an essential ingredient haemoglobin, as it is this that attracts th oxygen to the blood. When the supply iron is reduced, the number of red blo cells in the body is also reduced and th leads to a shortage of oxygen.

This deficiency is often the result eating the wrong foods, where the body simply not being fed sufficient quantiti of iron as part of the diet. It can also b caused by a severe blood loss. Women a particularly prone to this problem because of the amount of blood they lo each month during menstruation, a lo

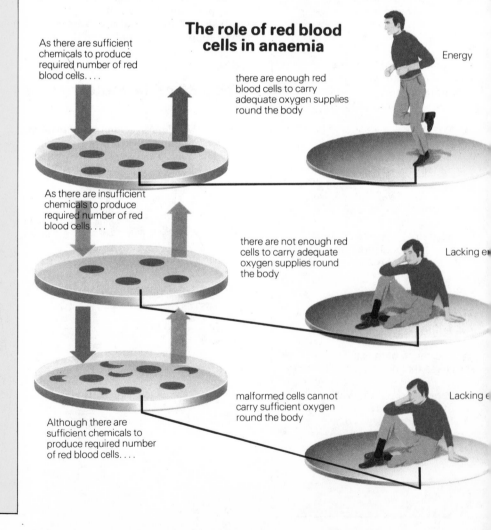

The role of red blood cells in anaemia

As there are sufficient chemicals to produce required number of red blood cells. . . .

there are enough red blood cells to carry adequate oxygen supplies round the body

Energy

As there are insufficient chemicals to produce required number of red blood cells. . . .

there are not enough red cells to carry adequate oxygen supplies round the body

Lacking e

Although there are sufficient chemicals to produce required number of red blood cells. . . .

malformed cells cannot carry sufficient oxygen round the body

Lacking e

Types of anaemia

Type	Causes	Treatment
Iron deficiency	Heavy menstrual loss; acute blood loss, bleeding duodenal ulcer; poor diet	Iron tablets or injections over several months
Pernicious anaemia	Failure of stomach lining to secrete substance called intrinsic factor	Vitamin B_{12} injections once a month for life
Anaemia of chronic diseases	Certain kidney diseases and some other chronic complaints	Anaemia usually disappears upon treatment of underlying disease
Aplastic anaemia	Bone marrow fails to make required number of red blood cells; can be brought about by cancer	Long-term; isolation; antibiotics and transfusions; drug treatment of marrow; marrow transplant
Sickle-cell anaemia	Defective red blood cells due to defective haemoglobin; genetic	If severe, transfusion; occasionally drugs
Thalassaemia	Defective haemoglobin; genetic	If severe, regular transfusions; occasionally removal of spleen (has no harmful effects)
Haemolytic (many types)	Red cells are killed off too early or in too great numbers in spleen	Drugs or removal of spleen, depending on type of anaemia

...at, if heavy, depletes the body of its ...ore of iron. The problem also occurs ...ring pregnancy when the mother loses ...on during the development of the baby.

Further iron deficiencies are caused by ...ptic ulcers, where there is a slow but ...eady bleeding, and by parasites such as ...ookworms and tapeworms which feed off ...e blood.

Another condition known as pernicious ...aemia occurs when the stomach lining ...ils to make and create a substance, ...naginatively (if somewhat, confusingly) ...alled intrinsic factor. This results in a ...eficiency of vitamin B_{12}, a vitamin that ...essential for the production of red blood ...lls. Since vitamin B_{12} can only be ...osorbed into the body with the help of ...trinsic factor, if its secretion comes to a ...alt, the number of red cells is reduced ...esulting in an anaemic condition.

Chronic diseases, such as rheumatoid ...rthritis and certain kidney diseases, ...ay also cause anaemia. The reason is ...ot yet completely clear, but it appears ...at the body's ability to utilize iron ...reaks down.

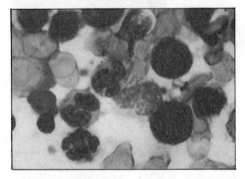

The larger, solid looking red blood cells in this bone marrow are typical of pernicious anaemia.

Instead of iron passing to the bone marrow, it is actually retained in the tissues. The resulting lack of iron in the marrow reduces the output of red blood cells.

A blood test used to diagnose the exact cause of the anaemia. A sample of blood is first collected from the patient (left) and then analyzed (right).

Perhaps the most serious form of anaemia is aplastic anaemia. This occurs when the bone marrow's ability to make red blood cells (as well as white cells and platelets – two further constituents of blood, both of which are made in the bone marrow) is arrested. Again, the cause is not fully known, but it does appear to be brought about by chemicals contained in some medicines or by cancer. This is a particularly unpleasant form of anaemia as not only do the body tissues lose their vital source of oxygen, but the body also loses the ability to ward off infection due to the lack of white cells.

There are many types of haemolytic anaemia, which occurs when the red cells are destroyed too quickly. It may occur either as a result of a blood transfusion mismatch or a complication with an Rh-negative mother. With some types of haemolytic anaemia there is a tendency to run in families.

There are further types of anaemia including those of a genetic and hereditary nature. Sickle-cell anaemia, common among black communities,

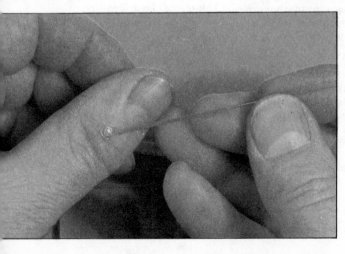

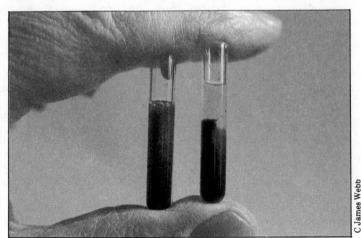

C James Webb

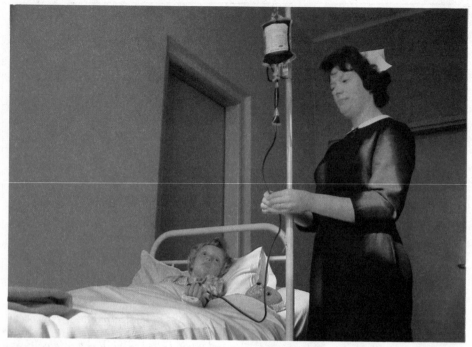

Zefa

If the anaemia becomes severe, a blood transfusion may be needed to ensure the necessary supply of oxygen to all parts of the body via the new blood.

arises through a malformation of the red blood cells, which fail to retain the necessary amount of oxygen. If the condition is severe, a blood transfusion may be necessary. Thalassaemia, common in Greek and other Mediterranean communities, is similar to sickle-cell anaemia. The haemoglobin is produced in an abnormal form.

Symptoms

To a great extent, the symptoms depend on the speed with which the anaemia develops, and this is influenced by the initial causes.

The most common symptoms are lethargy, pallor and breathlessness, sometimes accompanied by palpitations depending on the severity and type of anaemia. Severe cases of anaemia – such as those resulting from rapid loss of blood will cause fainting, dizziness and sweating. Symptoms of pernicious anaemia may also include 'pins and needles' in the hands and feet, nose-bleeds, and, in extremely severe cases, heart failure.

When children suffer from iron deficiency they may also show signs of irritability and hold their breath. In severe cases of iron deficiency, the usual symptoms may be accompanied by thirst, and some loss of control as the oxygen supply to the patient's brain is reduced.

Aplastic anaemia can develop slowly, becoming obvious only weeks or months after exposure to a poison. It has all the normal symptoms of anaemia but is also accompanied by infections due to the deficiency of white blood cells.

Prevention

Most types of anaemia are impossible to guard against as they result from a malfunction of the blood-making system. But steps can be taken to prevent the onset of iron deficiency anaemia. Eating a good balanced diet of milk, meat (especially liver), fresh fruit and vegetables, all of which contain an abundant supply of all those vitamins needed to make blood and which are also rich in iron, will contribute to good health and keep anaemia at bay.

The modern fad of taking tonics and vitamin pills is of little or no value unless recommended by your doctor, or you have difficulty following a balanced diet. However, because of the demands made on their systems, pregnant mothers may be advised by their doctors to boost their iron intake with iron tablets.

Dangers

It is most important that the origin of the anaemia is diagnosed as soon as possible for a quick return to full health. With most forms of anaemia the dangers are not immediate, but the condition can deteriorate progressively if left untreated.

However, in the case of acute blood loss, if the condition is not promptly controlled it may lead to a fall in blood pressure and, in extreme cases, the resultant reduction in oxygen supply may be a threat to the person's life.

Chronic anaemia may often worsen an already existing disease, and this is particularly true of elderly patients.

Anaemia can be particularly dangerous during pregnancy, as it will be passed on to the child. This will deprive the child of the oxygen so necessary for growth and development.

Treatment

Treatments vary according to the anaemia, but invariably the patient will be treated to counteract the initial symptoms while undergoing tests to discover the underlying cause.

Simple iron deficiency anaemia is normally treated with a course of iron tablets or injections, often lasting several months.

With pernicious anaemia, the missing B_{12} vitamin has to be given on a regular basis – usually once a month. And since the cause of the missing vitamin is the stomach's failure to secrete the intrinsic factor – a disorder that will never improve – the treatment lasts for life.

Anaemia of chronic disease can only be treated by resolving the underlying disease. Once this is done the anaemia will disappear.

The treatment for aplastic anaemia is usually long-term, the patient being treated in a special isolation unit designed to prevent infection. The treatment consists of giving antibiotics by drip to fight infection, and regular blood transfusions to keep fresh blood in circulation. The patient's bone marrow may be encouraged to recover with the use of certain drugs. In some cases, bone marrow transplants have been very successful as a treatment for this type of complaint.

Outlook

This depends very much on the type of anaemia and on the presence of an underlying disorder. In some cases, such as pernicious anaemia, improvement can sometimes be dramatic.

Iron deficiency anaemia is usually cured fairly promptly with the patient gradually gaining in strength and energy. But the underlying cause will still have to be treated by drugs, diet or surgery.

The outlook for the sufferers of aplastic anaemia is not so good and bone marrow transplants are not an automatic cure in every case.

Nor are drugs always successful. However, doctors are hopeful of an improvement in the next few years.

In some cases of haemolytic forms of anaemia hospitalization may be necessary, but most types respond well to medical treatment.

Anaesthetics

Q **I have heard that people can suddenly 'come round' on the operating table and know what is happening. Is this true?**

A Provided the patient remains in the deeper stages of general anaesthesia, there is no 'coming round', although it is possible that the patient may dream that this is happening. Where an intravenous injection is used as the method of administering anaesthesia, it is possible for an unexpected 'coming round' to occur, but a skilled anaesthetist is always on guard against this.

Q **My aunt told me that she was so nervous about a recent operation that she had to be given an injection before leaving the ward for the operating theatre. Why was this?**

A This is quite usual and in no way out of the ordinary. All patients are usually treated to an appropriate 'cocktail' of drugs—called premedication—immediately before their operation. This makes the patients very drowsy and relaxed and also makes it much easier for the anaesthetist to do his job in the operating theatre.

Q **Like most people, I have secrets that I do not want made public. I am very worried that I may talk when under a general anaesthetic. Is it likely that I may give away something that I may later regret?**

A This is a common anxiety. When patients do mumble under anaesthesia, it is usually just dream-like nonsense. But in any case, the anaesthetist is a doctor and therefore bound by an oath of confidentiality with regard to whatever patients may say. So you have nothing to fear.

Q **Why do spinal anaesthetics work downwards and not upwards?**

A Quite simply, the answer is gravity. If, for some reason, it is found to be necessary to affect the spinal cord above the site of the injection, the patient can be tilted to make it effective.

Anaesthetics are among the miracles of modern medicine. They ensure that otherwise painful treatments and operations are virtually pain-free. But how exactly does anaesthesia work?

In the days before anaesthetics even the most minor operation could be agonizing —early cartoons of people having teeth drawn without anaesthetic are enough to convince anyone of how fortunate we are today.

Modern anaesthetics can be divided into several different groups according to how and where they act to reduce pain. They can be given to patients in a number of different ways.

General anaesthetics
These are used in treatments and surgery where the patient needs to be completely unconscious. They are always given by a qualified anaesthetist, a medical doctor

The patient, having been taken from the ward, is being given oxygen prior to the injection of a general anaesthetic into his hand, immediately before being taken into the operating theatre.

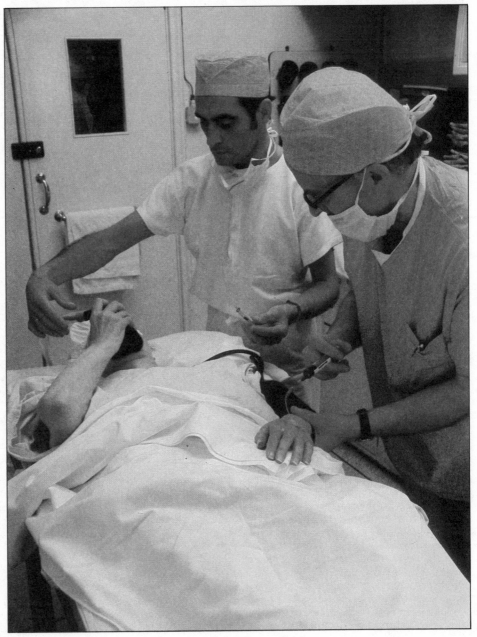

John Watney

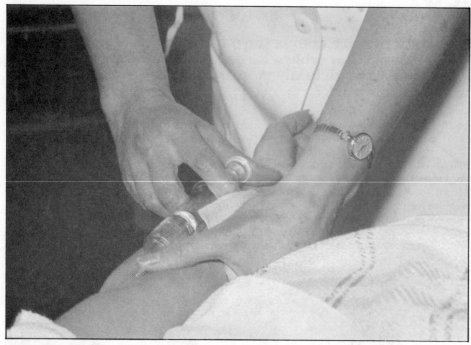

Ken Moreman

A general anaesthetic may be injected into a vein in the arm, as shown here, or into the back of the hand as shown on the previous page.

who has taken special training in the types and administration of anaesthesia. It is the anaesthetist's job to control the exact length of time during which the patient is to remain unconscious and to keep a careful watch on his or her physical condition.

They are given in one of two ways—either intravenously (injection into a vein) or by the patient's inhalation of a gas. Whether the injection is used on its own or combined with a gas at a later stage depends on the type and length of the operation.

Loss of consciousness may seem to occur quickly, but it is in fact a gradual process which happens in three different stages. In the first of these, the patient feels the pleasant sleep-like effects of the anaesthetic and starts to lose consciousness. This is the induction stage. The patient may feel extremely restless and talk aloud. During the second stage the patient is unconscious but still has some reflexes present and breathing is not quite regular. In the third and full stage of anaesthesia, the patient is fully unconscious with quiet regular breathing and relaxed muscles. The anaesthetist is trained to recognize the physical signs shown by the patient at each stage and ensure that any necessary action is taken. This continual monitoring is helped by the use of extremely sophisticated equipment in the operating theatre.

Many anaesthetic gases have been developed over the past 15 years, all of which are pleasant-smelling and ensure a quick return to consciousness.

When a general anaesthetic is given, muscle relaxants are also injected at the same time. Their purpose is to ease the way into the anaesthetized state—and when muscles are relaxed medical investigations or surgery are much easier to carry out.

Local anaesthetics

These can be rubbed on the area in the form of ointment or swallowed—if an internal anaesthetic is needed—in the form of a gel. They can also be sprayed but perhaps the most usual way in wh they are given is by injection, and ma people are familiar with this use in den treatment. They act by deadening nerves in the area so that pain messa do not reach the brain.

They produce a numbing, freezi effect so that a surgeon can operate wh the patient is fully conscious. The m widely used of the modern lo anaesthetics is called lignocaine; it can used in a variety of ways, but bupivaca is a newer preparation with a long lasting action; this can be injected and used as a spinal anaesthetic (an epidur in childbirth.

Pain relief in childbirth

An epidural anaesthetic is injected i the epidural layer of the spine in t lower part of the back to numb a lar area below the level of the injection. affects the nerves which link the spir cord and the womb, preventing pain m sages from being transferred along t spinal cord to the brain. The needle is l in place, strapped to the woman's bac until the baby is born so that repeat doses can easily be given when necessa This enables a woman to give birth pai lessly while still conscious and able co-operate where necessary, which essential in childbirth. Epidurals are a used in gynaecological operations and,

This inhaler allows the mother to breathe gas at her own rhythm to lessen the pain c contractions during labour. The gas is a mixture of one-half nitrous oxide and on half oxygen.

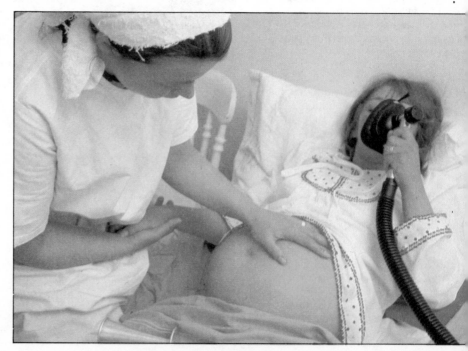

Types of anaesthetic

Anaesthetic	Effect	How given	Time needed to act
General	Complete loss of consciousness	Two methods: *Intravenous*—injection through a vein, usually at elbow or in hand (for shorter surgical or dental operations) *Inhalation*—given as gas through a mask (for longer operations or to maintain intravenous anaesthesia)	Rapid loss of consciousness. If patient told to count to 10—usually 'out' by number 7
Local	'Freezing' or numbing of particular area, e.g. gum and teeth in dentistry	Applied by spray or swab Made up in solution for injection or as drops As a gel or ointment	On surface—almost immediately Under skin—within minutes
Spinal (An epidural)	Gives pain relief without loss of consciousness — for childbirth, gynaecological or spinal operations	Injected into epidural layer of spinal canal	In minutes
Obstetric	Pain relief in childbirth without loss of consciousness. Slight drowsiness	Inhaled through mask held in hand. Automatically dropped when too drowsy	Only momentary loss of consciousness

Stages of general anaesthesia

Pre-medication	Stage One	Stage Two	Stage Three
A sedative injection is given to calm and relax patient while still in hospital ward. Can be combined with muscle relaxant injection	Pleasant sleep-like effect Loss of consciousness begins Some restlessness and talking aloud (Stage One is reached with gas and air pain relief in childbirth)	Patient is unconscious but reflexes still present Breathing not quite regular	Patient is fully unconscious Breathing is quiet and regular Muscles relaxed

some cases, it is used in the treatment of severe back problems.

There are other forms of pain relief available to women who decide not to have an epidural. To ease a painful contraction during labour, a woman can inhale gas and air (nitrous oxide with oxygen gas) using a vaporizer (a mask) which she holds in her hand. If she becomes too drowsy, she will automatically release the vaporizer; in this way she can have pain relief without completely losing consciousness.

For more difficult problems in childbirth, or for Caesarean birth, there are many modern general anaesthetics which can be used freely without risk either to mother or child.

Dental uses

Today, giving general anaesthetics during dentistry is losing popularity because of a number of fatal accidents which may have resulted because the dentist did not have the essential help of an anaesthetist. Any treatment requiring a general anaesthetic should be carried out in hospital—and many people now have their wisdom teeth removed under a general anaesthetic in hospital rather than in a dental surgery.

Local anaesthetics given by injection are still the most usual form of painkiller given, but many dentists are turning increasingly to the use of tranquillizers, such as Valium, especially in the case of more nervous patients.

After-effects

There are relatively few after-effects nowadays. With local and spinal anaesthetics, a little aching at the site of the injection may be felt for a few hours. In the case of general anaesthetics, the nausea and sickness that once occurred so frequently is now unusual. There may be some feeling of drowsiness, however, so that people who have had out-patient treatment or dental extraction should not drive a car immediately afterwards, and it is a wise precaution to see that there is someone to see them home.

Mild jaundice can occur, but this is a rare reaction to a general anaesthetic which should always be reported to the doctor immediately.

Anorexia nervosa

Q Sometimes I feel like going out and splurging on a bag of cream buns. Then I'm sorry, so I make myself sick afterwards. Am I anorexic?

A Not according to the actual definition of this illness. But watch out. You obviously feel guilty about overeating. Try to be less emotional about it and attempt to lose weight in a more sensible way.

Q Can anorexia occur in an older woman?

A Very occasionally. It is usually associated with immaturity, a fear of growing up, or the desire to revert to a child-like state, physically and mentally.

Q Are parents to blame for anorexia in a girl?

A Not in the deliberate sense. Girls with this problem often have very loving and protective parents. But sometimes this can be so repressive it stunts the normal process of growing up.

Q Can a person really die from slimming?

A Yes, if this turns into anorexia nervosa—from which about a quarter of the victims die. Fortunately, increased understanding and earlier treatment of this condition can give a better chance of a cure.

Q My friend has been told that she is anorexic, but she doesn't believe it. Why can't she realize how emaciated she looks?

A Because part of the disease itself is an abnormal mental state. A sufferer will look in a mirror but not see herself as she really is.

Q How is it that my daughter seems to eat normally but still loses weight?

A She may be pretending to eat but actually smuggling food out in her pocket or handbag. Suggest she sees the doctor to rule out any other cause of losing weight. He will understand the potential danger and take the necessary steps.

When a girl starts dieting, there may be more to it than a desire to be slim. Allowed to go too far, it can develop into anorexia nervosa—a potentially fatal disease. So it is vital for parents to know how they can help.

Anorexia nervosa is commonly known as the 'slimmer's disease', but despite this description its cause is far more complex than any simple desire to lose weight. It is also far more compulsive in its effects than ordinary slimming or dieting.

It almost always strikes young people between the ages of 11 and 30, and it affects more girls than boys. Apparently those from better-off homes are more prone to it than those from less affluent ones. This tends to suggest that anorexia nervosa is very much more a problem of the developed world.

Dramatic loss of weight is the obvious sign that something is wrong, and the person may need hospital treatment if it has reached a really serious stage. But, in the long run, the underlying causes must be diagnosed and remedied if treatment is to work and any improvement in weight and health maintained.

Causes

Once rare, anorexia nervosa is now tragically on the increase. The parents of victims may find it difficult to understand its cause, but more often than not the problem lies within the family. A daughter who never rebels or gives trouble, who delights her parents in every way and seems part of a perfect family, may

Teenage anorexics are often devious enough to hide food—something parents must be on their guard against.

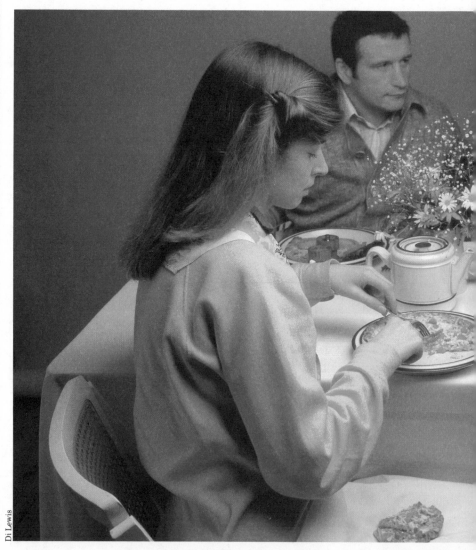

Di Lewis

cretly be tortured by a basic lack of
nfidence, self-esteem and a true idea of
erself as a person. She may be too sub-
issive and anxious to please for her own
ood. Her parents may have unwittingly
een the cause of this situation by being
ver-protective, thus deterring her
ormal adolescent drive towards in-
ependence and a separate identity.

Behind such a girl's unexpressed feel-
gs of inadequacy may lurk deeper and
orse fears of the demands that maturity
ay bring. These can lead to thinness
eing seen as a desirable goal.

If body fat is made to disappear and a
eutral childish figure retained, then the
roblems of adult life will not have to be
ced. The popular image of slimness and
perficial prettiness that is promoted by
lms, advertising and television may
ive a girl exactly the justification for
hich she is looking to account for her
ejection of food. In fact, she may not be
verweight at all.

Other girls diet drastically to increase
eir sexual confidence. These girls can

How to tell if your child is at risk

Appearance	Physical signs	Behaviour
Haggard face	Periods cease	Hypersensitivity about appearance
Stick-like limbs	Diarrhoea, alternating with constipation	Food binges, followed by vomiting
Obvious loss of weight	Vomiting	Smuggling food away; pretending to eat
Clothes too big	Cold skin	Undue interest in and purchasing of laxatives, emetics, diuretics and enemas
		Bad results from school
	Poor circulation	Anti-social acts, e.g. stealing or deliberately breaking things
	Liability to infection	Withdrawal from friends

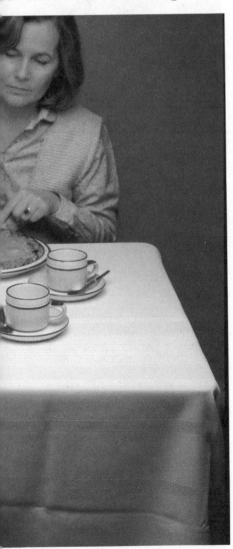

obstinately cling to the distorted idea
that their extreme emaciation is beautiful, ignoring the harrowing evidence to
the contrary which is only too obvious to
everyone else.

Dangers
Experience has shown that the more distorted an idea the victim has of herself,
the more difficult the cure, and the longer
the condition goes untreated the more uncertain the outcome. In the past, death
rates of between five and 25 per cent have
been reported, but better understanding
of the causes may improve the situation.

Anorexia nervosa must never be
lightly dismissed as a passing fad or
phase, which time and maturity will
cure. The anorexic is *not* mature, nor is
she suddenly likely to become so. Spontaneous cures rarely happen because the
victim takes a positive pride in sus-
taining her hunger strike.

The longer the illness lasts and the
more weight that is lost, the greater the
sense of achievement. This deepens in the
anorexic the illusion that being thin is
making her significant and outstanding
as an individual. In more real terms it is
also succeeding in focusing attention and
at last providing a form of personal rebellion against parental authority that
should have been made much earlier—
and in a less dangerous form—as part of
growing up.

Compulsive dieting
When a normal person embarks on
drastic dieting they can stop when they so
choose. Most find it so unpleasant to be
hungry or deprived of favourite foods in
the midst of plenty, that the real problem
is keeping to the diet. But the anorexic,

once set on a course of self-starvation,
cannot go into reverse. It is as though
they are the victims of a feeling not unlike that imposed by alcohol or drugs—
and with something of the same light-
headedness.

It has been suggested that anorexics
may even have a different body chemistry, but this has never been proved. It
seems far more likely that they simply
have a different mental outlook and confused motives that can involve not only
self-punishment but also punishment of
their parents.

Symptoms
It is vital that the illness is recognized
and that treatment started as early as
possible. This is not easy in the initial
stages until the weight loss becomes so
obvious that it is clear that something is
severely wrong and a visit to the doctor
really necessary. An unmistakable
symptom in a girl, once weight has fallen
below 46kg (103 lb) or thereabouts, is
that her periods stop.

It may be discovered that she is making
herself vomit, either to get rid of food she
has been coaxed to eat or as part of a
'binge-and-vomit' pattern, enabling her
to indulge in food without putting on the
detested weight. In the end, the body
becomes so accustomed to existing on a
greatly reduced amount of food, that it
has difficulty in coping with a large meal.

In a few cases, anorexics use emetics,
laxatives, diuretics and even enemas,
and over a period of time they can badly
disturb body chemistry and greatly increase the risk of a fatal outcome.
Obviously, prolonged starvation can
mean a general weakening in victims and
a greater susceptibility to infection.

Q My new boyfriend says that I'm too fat! In fact, I've always tended to be overweight and would like to do something about it—but I'm worried that I might overdo things and even develop anorexia nervosa and become really ill.

A Anorexia nervosa is not something that you catch, or that steals up on you in the night! Although it is the result of excessive or crazy dieting that pays no attention to the body's basic needs, it is fundamentally due to a disordered state of mind with regard to weight in particular and the rest of life in general. If you use a scientifically worked out diet—one that will enable you to lose weight but that still ensures that you get enough of all the food substances that your body cannot do without—you will never be in danger of getting anorexia nervosa. And you will be able to become as slim as you decide is best for you in perfect safety!

Q My grandmother, who is seventy-two, was in hospital recently for some tests and overheard the specialist say to his students that she had anorexia. I thought that this only happened to people of my age or am I completely wrong?

A There is a confusion of terms here. The anorexia you have in mind, which most commonly occurs in adolescent girls and which has been very much on the increase in recent years and consequently very much on people's minds and in the news is strictly speaking called anorexia nervosa, although it is often referred to as anorexia for short. But anorexia as a medical term has been around for centuries. It means loss of, or poor, appetite and is usually accompanied by loss of weight—and it was most likely this that the specialist meant when he was discussing your grandmother's case with his students.

Anorexia is an important feature in many conditions such as alcoholism, anxiety states and cancer. These possibilities are all carefully considered by the doctor when a case of suspected anorexia nervosa is being investigated to determine the best treatment.

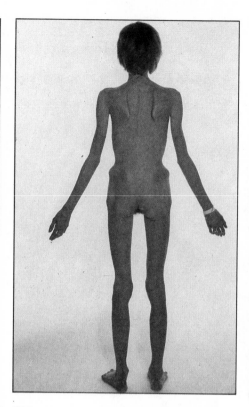

This anorexic girl, aged nineteen, was admitted to hospital and placed under treatment.

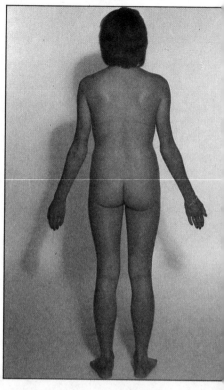

Two months later, she had returned to her normal body weight and had established good eating habits.

Treatment

Alert families should call for medical help long before symptoms are acute. The first job is often to restore weight to at least above danger level, before psychiatric treatment can commence. American research on this condition suggests that there is a critical weight which must be achieved, between 41 and 43 kg (90 and 95 lb) before psychotherapy can penetrate the strange mental isolation that starvation imposes and allow real communication to take place.

Weight gain for the anorexic often requires a prolonged stay in hospital, with intravenous feeding in the early stages. To coax the patient gradually to eat normal food and gain a set amount of weight, a system of rewards and withdrawal of privileges has been widely used. The basis for rewards is often a list drawn up by the patient and includes such things as being allowed to get up to go to the toilet, having extra visitors, wearing day clothes, going home on leave or, finally, going home altogether.

Maintaining a successful weight increase at home is made difficult by the extreme cunning of anorexics, who will use fair means or foul to avoid eating. They will deceive parents into believing they are eating a main meal at school or at work, and at home will toy with food, pretending to eat while secretly smuggling it from the table in pockets or handkerchiefs. They have even been known to fake a weight gain on the scale by putting weights in their pockets.

In a hospital ward, of course, this type of deception is less easy; weight is monitored and bed rest imposed. Also, in the early stages, a tranquillizer may be used. This will be given intravenously, if necessary, for those patients who know how to induce vomiting when given drugs or food by mouth.

Future action

Once enough weight has been gained for the patient to be out of immediate danger the more difficult part of the treatment can begin. This will include some family counselling, so that parents can understand the nature of the illness and its causes and so learn to cope with it.

Initially, the victim has to be convinced that anorexia nervosa is not just a matter of weight loss. The girl, helped by the therapist, can then begin her own search and fight for identity, dealing with the inner doubts and fears that plagued her, accepting the challenges and appreciating the real promise of her own sexuality and maturity. She must be helped to realize that her old ideas about herself were distorted and to replace them gradually with a truer picture. With this will come the self-confidence to grow up.

Antibiotics

C. James Webb

Ken Moreman

Q **Why doesn't my doctor prescribe an antibiotic when I get a sore throat, cold or cough?**

A Because antibiotics are not likely to be effective against them. These drugs only work on diseases caused by bacteria. Colds, 'flu and most sore throats are carried by viruses, a different type of germ.

Q **There are some old antibiotics in the medicine cupboard. Can I take them for the same problem as I took them for last year?**

A No. Never take old antibiotics, or capsules prescribed for someone other than yourself. It could be dangerous. Always consult your doctor.

Q **I am on the Pill. Will I have problems if I take an antibiotic?**

A Most antibiotics do not affect the action of the contraceptive Pill, but one, called rifampicin, destroys the Pill in the body, making it ineffective. Another, ampicillin, makes the Pill less effective. So you should always remind the doctor that you are on the Pill.

Q **Can I drink alcohol while I am on antibiotics?**

A Most antibiotics have no ill-effects when combined with alcohol. Warnings about use with alcohol are almost always printed on the container in which the antibiotic is packed. In any event, your doctor will almost certainly advise you on this at the time he prescribes them for you.

Q **Can antibiotics be taken during pregnancy?**

A No drug should be taken during pregnancy unless it is essential for the mother's well-being. At present we have no certain way of testing whether drugs are safe for the unborn child. Although much animal testing is carried out, this does not give reliable information about human safety. Tetracyclines taken during pregnancy can cause discolouration in the teeth of a child. Your doctor will be well aware of the dangers and will advise you.

Antibiotics fight a great variety of infections and have conquered or controlled many widespread and deadly diseases. So how do these 'miracle drugs' work?

Being prescribed a course of antibiotics is such a common experience today that many people have forgotten that these drugs have made possible some of the most dramatic advances of modern medicine, and, of course, saved countless lives.

The first antibiotic, penicillin, was introduced in the 1940s. Since then the search for, and discovery of, new types has been almost continuous, and the various antibiotics have between them dramatically reduced the mortality rates from several of the world's severe diseases.

Life savers

Because of antibiotics, pneumonia is no longer a killer. The venereal diseases, syphilis and gonorrhoea, can be cured if detected early enough. People who catch typhoid usually need not fear for their lives. Sufferers from bronchitis, that persistent and distressing chest infection, can be helped considerably. Deaths from meningitis, an inflammation of the membranes which envelop the brain and spinal cord, are much fewer than they ever were.

Antibiotics are also used to combat infection in patients who have undergone surgery, or those with serious body wounds. Again, the number of lives saved is substantial.

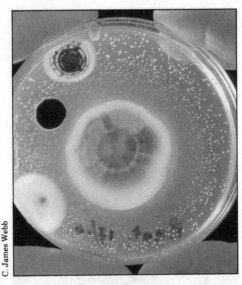

Above: Penicillin mould being cultured under laboratory conditions to produce an effective drug.
Right: Penicillin allergy rash.

And these drugs also cure many relatively minor problems such as throat infections, tonsillitis, cystitis (the urinary problem) abscesses, carbuncles, and septic fingers.

What they can do

Most of the time, we are exposed to what doctors and scientists call micro-organisms—in other words, germs. They are in food, in the air we breathe, in plants, the soil and in our own bodies. Most are harmless to human beings, many are beneficial, but a few are not and these cause disease.

Micro-organisms which cause disease are divided into a number of different types. Perhaps the three most commonly encountered are bacteria, viruses and protozoa. They all attack the body in different ways to cause different illnesses. Among the many conditions caused by bacteria are pneumonia and tuberculosis. Viruses cause such ailments as the common cold, flu, chicken pox, and smallpox. Protozoa bring about, among other things, amoebic dysentry and vaginal irritations.

Antibiotics are, quite simply, drugs which kill bacteria. They have no effect on viruses, are not prescribed for them, and, strictly speaking, are not used against protozoal infection either.

How they work

Antibiotics can be thought of as actually attacking micro-organisms, breaking them down and preventing their growth and multiplication within the body.

The most remarkable part of antibiotic action is that it is selective. This means that a given antibiotic drug only works on certain types of micro-organism, literally 'homing in' on the foreign bodies they are intended to kill, and leaving the other bacteria in the body unharmed.

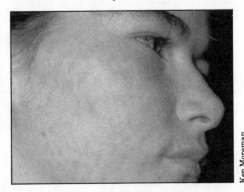

Antibiotics and their uses

Antibiotic	Uses
Penicillins The best-known, most widely used group. Common types: Penicillin G (usually injected), Penicillin V tables, Ampicillin capsules, Amoxicillin capsules and Talampicillin tablets	Some forms of tonsillitis, pneumonia, meningitis, syphilis, gonorrhoea, cystitis urinary infections, septic fingers, bronchitis, carbuncles
Tetracyclines A group of antibiotics developed after penicillin which considerably widened their effective range. Common types, usually taken by mouth, are Tetracycline itself, Oxytetracycline and a combination of the two	Infections of the respiratory (breathing) system; urinary infections; acne; rosacea (red nose); soft tissue infections such as some serious infections of the bones and sinuses
Erythromycin Common types, usually taken by mouth, are Erythrocin, Erythroped and Ilosone **Cotrimoxazole** Common types, taken as tablets, are Bactrium and Septrium	Respiratory infections; soft tissue infections Urinary infections and bronchitis Serious infections, especially of bones and sinuses
Cephalosporins The most recently developed group—originally discovered in a sewage effluent on the Mediterranean island of Sardinia. Chemical names include cephalexin and cephaloridine	Respiratory, genital, urinary, soft tissue and ear infections
Miscellaneous There is a large number of antibiotics of various types which are used more rarely. These include Chloromycetin, Streptomycin, Doxycycline, Gentamycin and Lincomycin	Each has a wide variety of types and may be effective in typhoid, meningitis and tuberculosis

Sulphonamides, which pre-date penicillin, are not actually antibiotics, but similar in action in that they fight bacteria and may be used against some infections for which antibiotics are also used. Some anti-protozoals, such as metronidazole (flagyl) are linked with antibiotics, but they are not, strictly speaking, the same.

To fully understand why antibiotics should be capable of this requires considerable specialist knowledge of chemistry. The basic theory, however, is fairly simple to understand. In nature, some micro-organisms just happen to attack and destroy others.

That this should be so was discovered by accident. The famous pathologist, Alexander Fleming, who discovered penicillin, noticed (as others had done before him without taking their findings any further) that certain bacteria stopped growing when placed close to the fungus called penicillium, most commonly found on mouldy bread.

The most active part of the penicillium fungus had then to be isolated to produce an effective antibiotic drug. With this knowledge of the chemical substances which kill micro-organisms, researchers could then move on to the next stage: copying them to produce artificial antibiotics. So now they are mostly produced artificially.

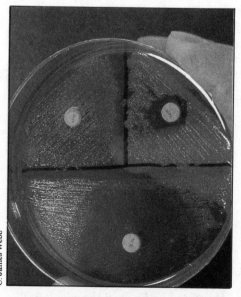

C. James Webb

Penicillin (centre each section) acting against different bacteria. Dark areas show strongest effects.

The fact that antibiotics oc[c]ur naturally has meant that new ones ha[ve] been discovered in what may seem to [be] extraordinary places. One, for exampl[e], was isolated from substances growing [on] dungheaps. But penicillin antibiotics [re]main to this day the most widely use[d].

Drawbacks

When antibiotics home in on bacter[ia] some will survive the attack, and, [re]markable though it may seem, 'lea[rn]' from the experience how to resist simi[lar] action in future.

The more an antibiotic is used, t[he] greater the number of bacteria learn [to] survive attack—in other words, build [up] 'resistance'.

So, in theory, antibiotics should be us[ed] as little as possible. If a bacteria becom[es] resistant to a certain antibiotic, as ha[p]pened, for example, with the first pe[ni]cillins, an alternative antibiotic has to [be] used. Luckily, the development of alt[er]native and synthetic antibiotic typ[es] means that this is possible. This is o[ne] reason why researchers are continual[ly] developing new types.

Side-effects

Some people are allergic to penicill[in,] usually coming out in a rash when giv[en] it. They should always tell anyone w[ho] treats them medically if this is the case[.]

Many antibiotics can have side-effec[ts] ranging from indigestion and diarrho[ea] to deafness and loss of balance. In mo[st] cases, it is a question of temporary d[is]comfort to be tolerated for the sake of [a] permanent cure. However, you shou[ld] always go back to your doctor witho[ut] delay if an antibiotic is having a pe[r]sistent, worrying side-effect.

Antibiotics really are 'miracle drug[s]' but like all precision instruments, the[y] need to be used properly. Medically, th[is] means tailoring the drug to the patient[s] infection. Bronchitis, or urinary pro[b]lems may, for example, be caused by on[e] bacteria in one attack, and a slight[ly] different one the next. Each needs [a] particular antibiotic to treat it.

The side-effects of taking a wron[g] antibiotic can in some cases be very u[n]pleasant, even dangerous. If you a[re] being treated by a new doctor—especial[ly] abroad—tell him if you know of a[n] antibiotic, or any other drug, that di[s]agrees with you. Never take anyone else[s] antibiotics. Never take antibiotics give[n] to you for a previous illness. Alwa[ys] complete a course of antibiotics give[n] you: if you do not, the bacteria have [a] greater chance of 'learning' how to be[come immune, and the infection could ge[t] worse. Never take antibiotics withou[t] being supervised by a doctor.

Anus

Once all the goodness has been extracted from the food we eat, the unwanted residue is excreted via the anus. But this is a sensitive area where irritating or painful disorders can occur; fortunately, these usually respond well to treatment.

Q Is it true that eating curry makes the anus itch?

A Eating highly spiced food such as curry can provoke an irritation of the anus because of the spices in the feces passing through the anal canal. If this is a problem, then avoidance of spicy food is the best cure.

Q The last couple of times that I have been to the toilet, I have noticed blood on the toilet paper. Could this be serious?

A It is always wise to consult your doctor if you notice blood in your feces or on the toilet paper or experience any bleeding from the anus. The underlying problem, when finally diagnosed, may well be a minor one, but it is not worth taking any risks.

Q My baby has diarrhoea and a rash has developed round his anus. What should I do?

A Diarrhoea can cause a rash to develop in the anal area due to continual irritation. To clear it up quickly, change the baby's diapers as soon as they become dirty and clean the affected area thoroughly with mild soap and water. Then dress the area with antiseptic cream or zinc ointment. Fresh air is also an effective healer, so it is a good idea to allow your baby to play for a while without a diaper on.

Q I am sometimes woken up in the night by an intense pain in my anus and back passage, but it seems to have nothing to do with passing feces. What is the cause, and should I see a doctor?

A The type of fleeting pain has the odd-sounding medical name of proctalgia fugax and is thought to be caused by spasms of the muscles in the lower part of the alimentary canal. It appears to be brought on by anxiety. The best way to deal with the pain is to get up and have a glass of water, or a hot drink. The pain should gradually subside. If it persists, occurs frequently or is adding to your worries, then by all means you should discuss the matter with your doctor.

The anus or anal canal is the very last section of the digestive system. It is about 10 cm (4in) long and is the opening through which the body's solid waste products—known as feces—are excreted.

How it works

As the feces near the end of their journey down the intestines, they gradually harden as liquids are absorbed by the body and the solid waste is pushed into the rectum. At the end of the anus are two rings of muscle, known as the internal and external sphincters. Normally the two spincters keep the anus closed, but during defecation—the passing of feces—they relax to allow it to escape. The internal sphincter (which is under the control of the nervous system; senses the presence of the feces and relaxes, allowing them to enter the anal canal. The external sphincter is kept closed deliberately (a skill we learn in babyhood) until a convenient moment presents itself when the feces can be passed. To ease the passage of the feces from the anus, the tissue in the lining of the canal secretes a lubricating fluid called mucus.

Anal problems

Problems in the anus range from the wildly irritating to the extremely uncomfortable, and most people will at some time or other suffer from an anal irritation of some sort. However, anal problems are most common in childhood, pregnancy and from middle age onwards. To help prevent some of them, it is sensible to wash the area regularly with warm water and mild unscented soap; dry with a soft towel.

Difficulty in the passing of hard feces often results in other trouble. The lining of the anal canal is quite delicate and passing hard motions can tear the lining. Not only does this mean that infection can enter the wound—known as an anal fissure—but it can become extremely painful to defecate. Unfortunately, the problem is often difficult to deal with as the sufferer may try to hold back the feces to avoid the pain. This has the effect of hardening the feces even further and so worsening the situation. Usually the problem is treated with antibiotics for the infection and a laxative to soften the feces.

In the long term, the best way to prevent this problem, which can affect both adults and children, is to eat a diet rich in bran and roughage. This has the effect of speeding the passage of feces through the last part of the alimentary canal and makes the feces softer because there is less time available for water to be absorbed back into the blood vessels

The small pattern of cracks in this anus are called fissures and are usually caused by passing a hard or very large, awkward stool. Because of constantly repeated irritation (further motions), fissures do not heal easily.

The development of a boil in the anus can lead to a fistula. The boil bursts but does not usually drain into the anus. Instead, drainage channels form through the skin and open to the outside of the body beside the anus.

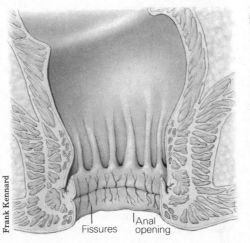

Fissures | Anal opening

Frank Kennard

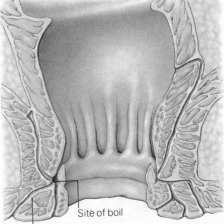

Site of boil

Fistula

Common causes of pain in the anal area

Symptoms	Possible cause	Action
Sharp pain during bowel movement and pain or aching for up to an hour afterwards; bleeding from anus	Anal fissure	Apply soothing ointment; have a warm salt bath for temporary relief; see a doctor. A lubricant may be prescribed and surgery recommended to remove the affected tissue and stretch the anal opening
Soreness not made better or worse by defecation; discharge from anal region.	Anal fistula	See a doctor. Antibiotics will be prescribed; an operation may be needed
Severe, throbbing pain	Abscess or boil	See a doctor. The pus will need to be surgically drained
Intense pain, not worse on passing feces; anus painful to touch, may itch; painful deep purple protrusion may appear on one side of anus	External piles	Apply ice cold water on a tissue or have a hot bath for temporary relief; see a doctor. Long term, take more exercise; eat more roughage; surgery may be needed
No pain but itching, soreness and the passage of much mucus; bright red blood may be lost on defecation; feeling of fullness in anus	Internal piles	See a doctor. An injection will provide temporary relief but surgical treatment will probably be needed
Pain may be worse on defecation; protrusion of pink tissue from anus	Prolapse (dropping) of rectum	See a doctor. An operation will probably be necessary, but in the case of a child the doctor may be able to push the collapsed part back into place

lining the canal. And a high roughage diet is helpful in preventing other anal problems such as piles and some disorders of the large intestine.

Further disorders
The most well-known of anal problems is piles (haemorrhoids). These are caused by abnormalities of the blood vessels surrounding the anal canal, forming clumps of swollen, contorted varicose veins both inside and outside the anus. According to their position piles are thus known as internal or external. They are extremely

In a prolapse, the muscles surrounding the rectum become weakened so that during defecation part of the rectum collapses and protrudes from the anus. To solve this problem the rectum may need stitching back into place.

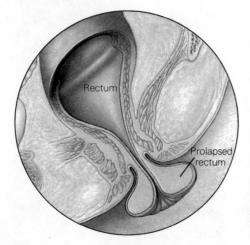

uncomfortable, cause irritation and itching, and are often accompanied by bleeding. Happily, if suppositories fail the piles can now be treated with injections or by surgery, if the condition is severe.

In children
Children are often susceptible to irritations around the anal opening and in younger children this is usually caused by diaper rash. Another anal irritation which is more common in children than adults is caused by threadworms—a type of parasite that lives in the lower bowel—and these cause severe itching around the anus, but can be treated with drugs.

In adults
In adulthood, constant itching of the anus—known as pruritius ani—can be caused by infection of the skin around the anus or by severe anxiety. Scratching the area can result in considerable skin damage, causing the infection to spread and the area to bleed.

The best treatments are antiseptic ointments to kill the bacteria and calamine lotion to cool the inflammation. But a doctor should be consulted as itching and irritation can be associated with other anal problems. In any disease of the spinal cord the sphincteral muscles may be paralyzed, resulting in an inability to control excretion.

Boils and abscesses are the most common types of infection in the anal canal, and they can be very uncomfortable—abscesses particularly so. This is

because a bad abscess can form a drainage channel—called a fistula—that opens to the outside of the body next to the anus. The fistula takes the form of a small red spot from which fluid leaks. This complaint is normally treated with antibiotics, and, in severe cases, surgery.

Complications
A further complication can also arise through the weakening of the internal muscles that surround the rectum. This leads to the lining of the rectum dropping, a complaint called a prolapse. It is easily indentifiable as the lining can be seen protruding from the anal opening. The weakness may be present at birth or develop with old age, or it can be brought on by pushing too hard during defecation, by diarrhoea, whooping cough or during labour. The complaint should always be reported to the doctor who will either push the lining back into position or, if the problem is severe, he or she may find it necessary to secure the lining with a few stitches.

Unwanted growths may also protrude from the anus. These normally take the form of benign lumps of tissue called polyps and they are particularly common in young children. Warts and wart-like tumours called papillomata may also occur, especially in middle and old age. In both cases the doctor may recommend diathermy, in which the growths are burned off electrically. However, the presence of papillomata necessitates surgical removal because they can lead to cancer.

Anxiety

Q What is the most important thing I can do when I have an attack of anxiety?

A One of the most helpful things you can do is stop, take some deep breaths, relax and think about what is causing your attack. One of the commonest problems with anxiety is panic, so that a sufferer is not able to deal with his or her anxiety calmly.

Q Can I die of anxiety?

A In real life one doesn't die of anxiety, but it is possible to die of side-effects, such as a heart attack brought on by an anxiety-producing situation. But anxiety is a relatively minor problem and you should be able to cope with it fairly easily.

Q What if my doctor prescribes drugs such as tranquillizers or sleeping pills? Can I become addicted to them?

A Unfortunately yes, particularly the sleeping pills. It's all too easy to use drugs to become calm and, seemingly, to remove the symptoms and even the causes of anxiety. But they are really only useful for helping you to alter your behaviour pattern or re-learn how to cope with the things that cause your anxiety. But this can be done without drugs—by seeking professional help and through sheer willpower.

Q Am I the only person who suffers from anxiety?

A No, certainly not. Almost everyone suffers from anxiety at some time in their lives. This can be something as simple as an anxiety based on superstition, like fear of the number 13. There are organizations set up to help all forms of anxiety. Your doctor should have a list.

Q Can babies feel anxiety?

A Yes, frequently. Being hungry or left alone can be terrifying for an infant who cannot communicate verbally. Only the repeated experience of being comforted and cared for will create a feeling of trust and reduce anxiety.

It is perfectly normal to feel anxious from time to time, but intense anxiety which disrupts the sufferer's life needs professional treatment.

We have all felt anxious at some time, whether we call it feeling uneasy, on edge or uptight. It is perfectly natural to feel anxious and, in fact, to some degree it can have good effects such as toning us up for a big match or sharpening awareness for an interview or exam.

But some forms of anxiety are not as healthy as others. If you get mildly worked up before an exam, that can be beneficial. However, if you cannot sleep well the night before, or begin to sweat profusely and feel nauseated as you enter the examination hall, this is a more serious anxiety attack and if you find that this is part of a continuing pattern, you should seek help.

A child's anxiety is readily dispelled by the loving reassurance of his mother.

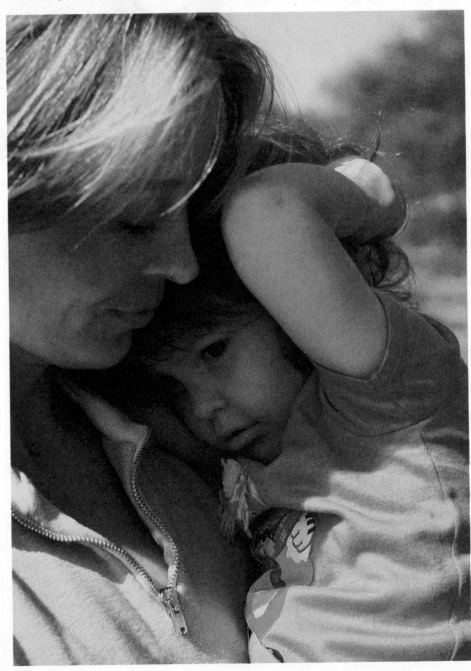

What is anxiety?

Our reaction to stress is an inbuilt survival mechanism that originally enabled us to act instantly when our lives were threatened. To prepare for action the heartbeat strengthens to pump blood to all the muscles, and blood pressure rises. Because the muscles need fuel to produce energy, blood sugar is released into the bloodstream and the oxygen required to turn this sugar into energy is taken into the lungs with quickened breathing, even gasping. Because the body has a limited supply of blood, some has to be diverted from other systems, so the blood supply to the stomach is reduced and digestion is disturbed. The mouth goes dry, the pupils dilate and, as the body overheats with increased blood supply to the muscles, the skin begins to sweat to cool it down. Adrenalin is released from the adrenal glands and keeps the stress reactions going.

When action has been taken and the danger is over or the problem resolved, the body relaxes and returns to normal once more. But when the threat is low-level and continuous as is common in the emotionally stressful situations of modern living, often no direct action can be taken to deal with it and the body will suffer the effects of long-term tension.

This is what is happening to the anxious person lying awake at 3 a.m. with a pounding heart and a stomach tied in knots over a purely emotional problem at work, for example. He is suffering from the same physical and chemical changes that were originally intended to save life, only now the reactions are inappropriate to the events.

Anxiety takes many forms. Some have obvious causes, as a fear of dogs in someone who was bitten or frightened by one as a child. Other forms are not so clear and may include anxiety about a relationship which can make you sexually impotent or frigid. Sometimes the cause of anxiety can be totally imaginary—a groundless fear that you are in line for the sack, for instance. Occasionally the anxiety takes an unspecific form, such as sudden, unexplained panic on the way to the office or a sense of general hopelessness about the state of the world (called 'angst').

Anxiety sufferers

Anxiety is experienced by both men and women, though women tend to seek help for it more than men. What is interesting is that there appear to be several times in life when people are more likely to suffer from anxiety.

The first of these times is the period of adolescence when young people are coming to terms with their own identi-

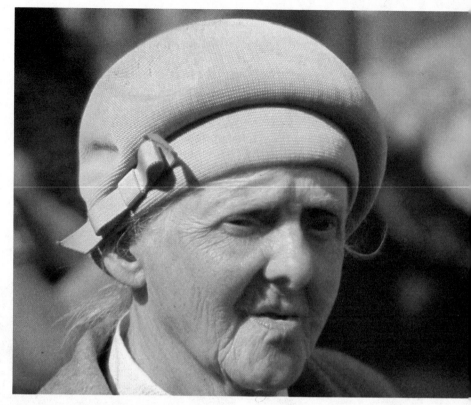

ties. Many of their anxieties are of a sexual nature or are an expression of the teenager's self-doubts.

This is aggravated by the need to be accepted by society based on its values—good looks, brightness, likeability—and also by the competitiveness among young people.

In the early thirties there is a new peak of anxiety. People begin to worry about success in their jobs and their incomes being sufficient for their needs. Men especially are concerned about whether or not they 'are going to make it to the top'. Marital conflicts, or potential ones, that could have been ignored or put aside in earlier years may come to the surface only now.

During their late forties or early fifties men and women tend to look back and perhaps feel a certain disappointment that they have not done better, or panic because there seems to be so little time left and so much still to accomplish. Because of hormonal changes at this time of life (part of the menopause, or 'change of life' when periods cease and the ability to bear children ends), women are especially vulnerable.

The later years of life can also bring new anxiety for both men and women. This is often related to loneliness and the feeling on the part of the older person that he or she is isolated from everyone else.

Dealing with physical and emotional 'growing pains' can be a source of anxiety.

Tension in the elderly may be caused by feelings of being isolated from others.

Causes

There are two main theories about the causes of anxiety. The first holds that it is due to a personality disorder that makes our psychological defences unable to work in the way they should. In other words, instead of recognizing the anxiety

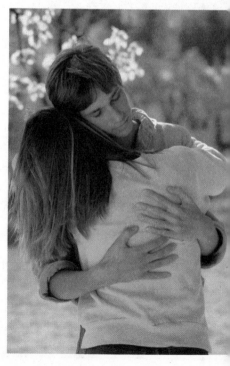

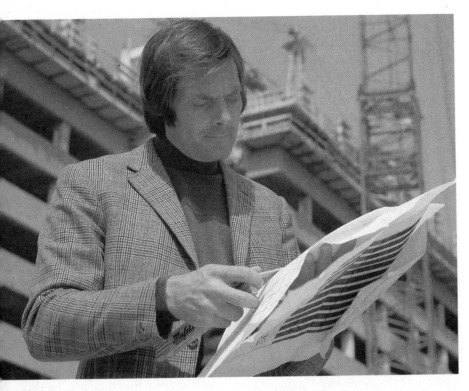

In their thirties people are prone to worry about success in their careers.

symptoms and dealing with them, the sufferer turns the symptoms into a pattern—one that is often self-destructive.

The second theory claims that there is a failure in some physical function, especially in the nervous system. This may be due to an imbalance of chemicals in the body. Supporters of this theory believe that these 'malfunctions' can be cured by effective and painless drug therapy.

Thirdly, some theorists suggest that the causes of the problem are much simpler than either of these theories suggest and that anxiety, in fact, is merely a result of modern life: the widespread loss of social and religious values and a response to conditions over which we no longer feel we have any control.

Symptoms

It can be said that anxiety is increased arousal about a particular event and that some people may become over-aroused when the specific trigger for their anxiety occurs, like a deadline that must be met. They then become over-excited and develop the physical symptoms associated with coping with an external threat: increased heartbeat, high blood pressure, excessive sweating, and rapid breathing resulting sometimes in giddiness or weakness at the knees.

Prolonged contraction of the muscles, readied for action, may cause cramp-like spasm, backache, the tender, aching spots in shoulders and neck so familiar to tense people, or headaches brought on by tensed forehead muscles or continually gritting the teeth. Digestive disorders may include spastic colon, indigestion, nausea, stomach cramps, and gastric ulcers. And because the digestive and urinary systems are 'working overtime', this may cause an endless number of visits to the toilet.

Other common symptoms are insomnia, chest pain, asthma, sexual difficulties, a lump in the throat or an inability to swallow, and migraine headaches, possibly precipitated by biochemical and physical changes in the body.

If the anxiety continues, secondary symptoms can develop; these can include skin rashes, spots, weight problems (under- or overweight). Strangely enough, those suffering from anxiety can also experience either increased aggression or the reverse effect, becoming completely inhibited, withdrawn and even extremely depressed.

The symptoms are unpredictable and the effects can be disruptive in everyday life. Though anxiety can occur at any time, attacks are more likely to be associated with a specific situation, like dealing with a marital problem, fear of the boss, learning a particular subject at school.

If the symptoms are bad, there will be a certain amount of discomfort, both physical and social—people are often not very understanding when others are suf-

Even a mild case of anxiety reveals itself in facial expressions and gestures.

fering from anxiety. But the worst effects are that some of the symptoms are physically weakening (such as inability to sleep which causes further complications like irritability) and, if they are bad, may prevent you participating fully in certain aspects of your life, as for example when spots or a rash occurs before an important event.

Treatment

It is possible to try and cope with anxiety on your own. The first thing to do is to recognize and accept the symptoms and try to discover and face the causes.

But, if this self-help process is not enough—even with the aid of family and friends—it is best for you to consult the doctor. He or she may refer you to a psychotherapist who will help you discover and cope with the causes. This treatment may be carried out either in individual sessions or in the company of other anxiety sufferers in group psychotherapy.

Many doctors are suggesting alternative therapies, the purpose of most of them being to help you relax and gain a greater self-awareness. These may include yoga, breathing exercises, biofeedback or even meditation.

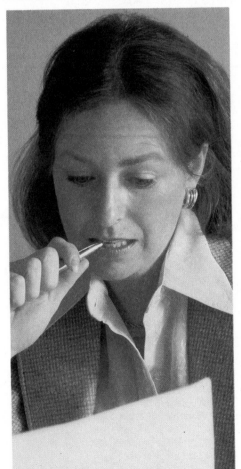

Aphasia

Aphasia is the loss of the ability to understand words and communicate through speech. It can be caused by injury or disease, but speech therapy can encourage recovery.

Q Does aphasia cause stuttering?

A A stammer is a disturbance of speech fluency, not due to brain damage or acquired defects in the speech centres. Both the bright and the slow child can develop it, and it is not at all a form of aphasia. But a speech therapist can help in the control and relief of a stutter.

Q I've heard it said that youngsters with brain damage to one side of the head will only suffer temporary aphasia, whereas adult aphasia is permanent. Why is this?

A In children *and* in adults aphasia may either be relatively temporary and improve rapidly or be more persistent. The difference lies more in the cause of the disturbance than in the age of the person with the disturbed language problem.

Q Is it true that the adult who speaks several languages fluently, and who develops aphasia is only left with speech of the original or 'mother tongue'?

A It does seem to be a feature of multilingual men and women who suffer strokes or injuries causing aphasia, that the vocabulary of foreign languages is lost or severely restricted. They have more of the 'mother tongue' left as a rule. As the aphasia improves, however, the other languages may return.

Q My mother has recently had a stroke and ever since seems to be speaking very slowly. Is this a kind of aphasia? Will it get better?

A Yes, it most probably is aphasia. Most stroke victims suffer this to some degree. It is difficult for them to both understand and to express themselves. For this reason, a great deal of patience is needed. They are just as frustrated as you are with the problem in communication, and impatience will not be of any help.

In most cases, the aphasia is a temporary condition and, given time, it will lessen. If there is no improvement in about two years, little is likely.

There are two important processes in the brain which control the power of speech. First, when a spoken message is received by the brain via the ears, the person is normally able to follow what is being said because the brain uses the memory to decode the sounds. Then, secondly, an answer is prepared. Ideas are turned into words (encoded), again using the memory to co-ordinate the process, and the muscles of the larynx (throat), jaw, lips and tongue are stimulated by the brain, enabling the person to speak and give the answer. These two processes take place in areas of the brain linked by nerves.

Receiving and decoding the spoken (and written) word takes place in the upper part of the right lobe of the human brain. When things go wrong here, the term used is sensory or receptive aphasia. Encoding the spoken word takes place in the left lobe of the brain, and upset or disturbance here is called motor or expressive aphasia.

Causes in adults

A range of diseases and conditions ca produce adult aphasia, but the co monest of these are complaints whi affect the flow of arterial blood to t speech centres of the brain. These inclu cerebral artery thrombosis (clotting cerebral artery haemorrhage and cer bral artery embolism (a foreign cl lodging in the blood vessels). They pr duce weakness in the limbs on the rig side of the body or paralysis (a 'strok and the aphasia accompanies the pow loss.

Head injuries which result from dor estic, road or works accidents or violer assault can also damage the centres speech causing sensory or motor aphasi or both together.

Rarer conditions affecting the brai such as cerebral tumours, cerebral de generation and damage following infec tion of the brain may sometimes produc forms of aphasia.

How the brain enables us to communicate

Words are heard (A); sound is received by primary auditory cortex (B), deciphered in Wernicke's area (C) and transmitted by nerves—arcuate fasciculus—(D) to Broca's area (E) where reply is formed and messag sent to face via motor cortex (F), which als stimulates muscles of lips, tongue, jaw and throat to produce speech.

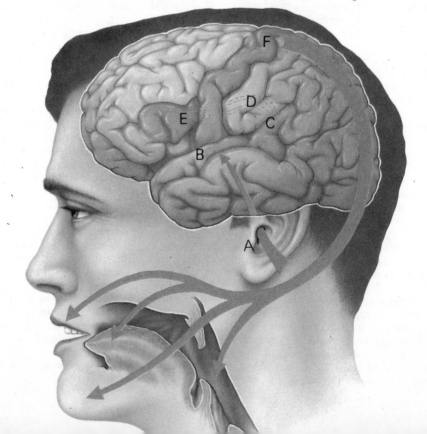

Types of adult aphasia

In the most severe form of adult motor or expressive aphasia, the individual may be left with only one or two words of expression, such as 'yes' or 'no', and even these may be used inappropriately. If there is no sensory or receptive aphasia, however, the motor aphasic person can still follow and understand speech and can carry out instructions.

This is important where the 'stroke' patient, for example, is being re-taught to use weak or paralyzed muscles and to carry out activities of daily living which restore his independence.

Severe motor aphasia is extremely frustrating for the sufferer since he or she cannot communicate thoughts and needs quickly and accurately. Writing, which is a form of motor language is unfortunately similarly affected.

In less severe forms, the person has more vocabulary, but it is still much less than he had before he became ill. He may tend to repeat fixed words or phrases in a stereotyped fashion, a form of aphasia called *palilalia*. His speech generally is hesitant and may be filled with more gaps than usual.

The least severe but still frustrating form of motor aphasia is *nominal* or *mnestic* aphasia. In this condition, the individual recognizes familiar objects but is unable to give them the appropriate names. For example, the person can demonstrate that a pen is an object to write with but cannot state directly that this is 'a pen'.

Another feature of some motor aphasic sufferers is that, although their ordinary vocabulary may be limited to a few words, they can still swear. There is no known medical reason for this.

Although the power to understand and follow the spoken word is limited or grossly disturbed in sensory or receptive aphasia, the person may speak quite fluently and noisily. The difficulty is that what is said may not make any sense to the listener because grammer and sound may be quite distorted, yet the speaker is unaware of this. This form of sensory aphasia is sometimes called *jargon* aphasia. Where the same nonsense phases are constantly repeated, this is described as *echolalia*.

Aphasia in children

Speech is a complex skill which children have to learn. For the skill to be mastered, the child's brain must function properly and the two speech centres must be intact. The child must be exposed to sounds and words, and must have the full articulation equipment, that is, the muscles of the jaw, face and larynx must co-ordinate properly.

Aphasia in children is therefore essentially a problem of speech learning and it can be caused by a range of handicaps, one or several of which may occur together. These include brain damage which may have happened before or during birth, spastic weakness, partial deafness, subnormal intelligence, and the condition known as autism (an emotional disorder in which the child completely withdraws from the real world, and is almost unable to communicate).

As well as showing symptoms of aphasia affecting adults, children also show other disturbances in their difficulties with words as symbols. There may be a failure to match the written and the spoken word. The child may try to read from right to left in a language normally read from left to right. Spelling words aloud or in spelling tests may reveal word difficulties. Parts of words may be moved around, creating bizarre results. Associated disturbances include the reading problem of dyslexia, or word blindness, and the writing problem of dysgraphia, or inability to form words.

Mothers generally notice speech delay and if this is pointed out to the family doctor or nursery school teacher, the child can be referred to a neurologist and an educational psychologist who can advise on possible improvement and recommend speech therapy or other training.

Treatment

The treatment of all forms of aphasia is nowadays undertaken by a qualified speech therapist, who works alongside the medical, nursing and physiotherapy staff where they are nursing a patient with a stroke or head injury.

To restore communication with the adult motor aphasic patient the therapist uses picture cards showing various common needs like food, toilet, washing or drinking, to which the patient can point. Alphabet cards and sheets may then be used which the patient can point to and use to construct words to get his message across. Stroke patients may be taught to write using the unaffected hand. Crosswords—spoken aloud—and tapes are also used as aids to speech recovery.

Strangely enough, the motor aphasic patient may sing quite fluently, even though speech is disturbed, and this can be used to communicate.

Family, friends and relatives can be helpful in talking to and encouraging the speech of the motor aphasic patient. Because of the patient's lack of ability to understand the treatment of severe sensory or receptive aphasia is difficult, but patients can sometimes be helped by the constant repetition of simple activities.

With motor aphasic children the aim is to teach speech instead of capitalizing on speech existing before illness. The speech therapist first does a 'language search' to find out how much language the young child has, then tries to enlarge this.

In treating an aphasic child, the speech therapist will first establish how much, if any, language the child already has and will then help to develop this.

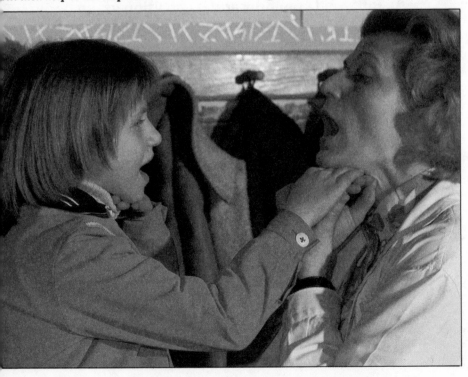

Appendicitis

Q I am a model for a swimwear firm and have to have my appendix out. Will I have an ugly scar afterwards?

A This rarely happens today. Various ways of sealing wounds have been devised which improve the cosmetic appearance of an operation scar. In any case, the scar from your appendix operation will be below the 'bikini line' so your job should not be affected.

Q Do people always pass wind after an appendix operation? I would be so embarrassed if this happened to me.

A Far from being an embarrassment, wind is a sign that the bowels are returning to life. After any abdominal operation, the bowels stop working for a while. In fact, food and drink cannot be taken until 'bowel sounds' return. The bowels are full of wind anyway, and as they gain strength, this is the first thing to be expelled.

Q My brother, who is a sailor, has a grumbling appendix. What would happen if it suddenly worsened while he was at sea?

A Obviously, if away from medical help, some treatment has to be tried, whether at sea or on a mountain top. Painkillers are essential and antibiotics may help. A large vessel may have a ship's doctor who is well qualified to deal with such an emergency; otherwise, modern communications are so rapid that air-sea rescue services can be called in to cope with any crisis that may occur.

Q I am planning a world trip and will undoubtedly visit places with no medical facilities. Since I have had attacks of appendicitis in the past, is it possible to have my appendix removed as a preventative measure?

A This is sometimes done, but not as a general rule. In the developed world the dangers of an unnecessary operation may outweigh the risks of sudden appendicitis. But in your case it may be a sensible precaution. Your doctor will be able to advise you.

The appendix is a small organ that was useful to our ancestors but is now virtually redundant. However, it can still cause trouble and sometimes has to be removed, but with modern surgical techniques, an appendectomy is both speedy and safe.

The appendix is a narrow, tube-like piece of gut resembling a tail, which is located at the end of the large intestine. The tip of the tube is closed; the other end joins on to the large intestine. It can be up to 10 cm (4 in) long and about 1.5 cm (5/8 in) in diameter.

It is only found in humans, certain species of apes and in the wombat. Other animals have an organ in the same position as the appendix that acts as an additional stomach, where cellulose, the fibrous part of plants, is digested by bacteria. It seems that as we evolved through the ages and began to eat less cellulose in favour of more meat, a special organ was no longer needed for its digestion. The appendix could therefore be described as a relic of evolution.

Appendicitis

Facts about the appendix appear to contradict one another. On the one hand, nature appears to have adapted it to act as a watchdog for infection at the lower end of the gut. Like the tonsils and adenoids, it contains a large collection of lymph glands for this purpose; but if the appendix does become inflamed, a condition called appendicitis results and the organ may have to be removed. On the other hand, the appendix seems by no means essential to health. It can be dispensed with at an early age, making no apparent difference, and has nearly shrivelled up completely by the age of 40 or so.

Appendicitis can occur at any time from babyhood to old age. However, it is rare under the age of two, more common among teenagers, and then becomes increasingly rare again over the age of 30. Why it should reach its peak in youth remains a mystery.

Causes

In fact, the history and incidence of the condition is extremely baffling. Up to the end of the 19th century, it was relatively unknown. This is still so in places like Asia, Africa and Polynesia. But in Europe, North America and Australia, for example, appendicitis is now a very common complaint.

The reason for this is thought to be directly related to changes in our eating

An inflamed appendix and its position in the body

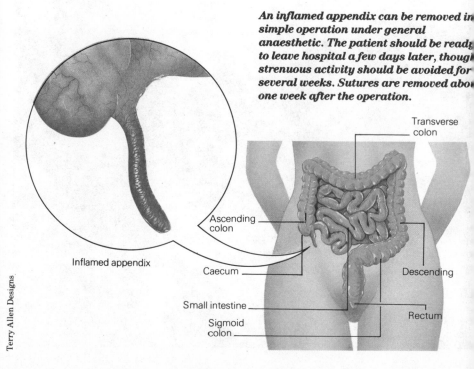

An inflamed appendix can be removed in a simple operation under general anaesthetic. The patient should be ready to leave hospital a few days later, though strenuous activity should be avoided for several weeks. Sutures are removed about one week after the operation.

Terry Allen Designs

Inflamed appendix

Ascending colon

Caecum

Small intestine

Sigmoid colon

Transverse colon

Descending

Rectum

abits. The modern western diet has become so refined that it now lacks ufficient fibre—called roughage. This eficiency causes the food to slow down in s passage through the intestines. This uggishness can lead to blockages, which ay be a cause of appendicitis. Food esidues can occasionally collect in the ppendix and form an obstruction. Pips, uit stones and other foreign bodies that ay have been swallowed accidentally an also aggravate the appendix, but hese are fortunately among the rarer auses of appendicitis.

Worms, the result of eating contaminated food, are another danger to the ppendix. These intestinal parasites may dge there and eventually cause an ostruction. Whatever their origin, lockages of any kind can lead to the nset of appendicitis.

he 'grumbling' appendix

ecurrent attacks of appendicitis, each asting a day or two, can sometimes occur. s the appendix gets inflamed, the intestines nearby close round it to wall off he infection. If the inflammation clears p, the intestines may still be left stuck round the appendix. These 'adhesions' an restrain the normal movement of food round the system, resulting in colicky griping) pains, which may then be felt in he appendix region during normal digeson. This gives rise to a 'grumbling' ppendix, which will settle if it does not ecome inflamed again.

erious symptoms

or various reasons, a bout of appenicitis may not clear up on its own: the ppendix is blocked and further action ill be necessary.

The early symptoms of appendicitis are ot easy to distinguish from any other orm of tummyache. Pain, which comes nd goes in a colicky fashion is felt round the umbilicus (tummy button), as he appendix muscles contract while rying to drive any obstruction out. If here is no obstruction, then there will ust be a constant ache.

After six to 12 hours, the symptoms vill change, as inflammation builds up round the appendix. The overlying perioneum (lining) of the abdomen becomes rritated and, as this is well supplied with erves, more pain is felt around the ppendix. Usually, this is in the right ower abdomen. However, the site of the naximum pain is variable.

Diagnosis

Often the patient has to press his or her wn stomach to establish where it hurts nost. The most common site is two-thirds f the way along a line joining the top of

Recognizing appendicitis

Early symptoms	Action
Colicky (griping) pain in stomach that comes and goes	Give mild painkiller e.g. acetaminophen
Loss of appetite	Try a soothing drink: warm milk or weak tea
Constipation	Give a hot water bottle
	DO NOT GIVE A LAXATIVE—this will be harmful, causing painful contractions of the appendix and increasing the chance of perforation
In children, a respiratory infection may show symptoms imitating appendicitis. These *could* be genuine	TELL THE DOCTOR ABOUT TUMMY SYMPTOMS IN CHILD—just in case

Later symptoms Give no more home remedies.
GET MEDICAL HELP AT ONCE

More pain in appendix area (right lower abdomen)	Patient lies with right leg flexed up. Stretching it down produces pain.
Pain may move up or down from umbilicus (tummy button)	Diarrhoea possible, but constipation more common
Slight rise in temperature e.g. 37.5°C (99.5°F)	Nausea
Slight increase in pulse rate	Vomiting
	Foul-smelling breath

Means of viewing the appendix

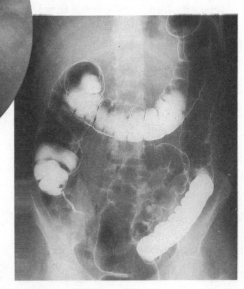

A normal appendix (above) as seen through an endoscope, a viewing instrument which is inserted in the abdomen and which can be used to take photographs inside the body. This is how a healthy appendix appears (right) when X-rayed.

Q A great-aunt of mine died of appendicitis. Could this happen nowadays?

A This is most unlikely. In the past, any operation was fraught with dangers. As a result, an appendix operation was often delayed until perforation occurred and the patient would then become rapidly ill and even die.

Q Several members of my family have had to have their appendix out. Is this just a coincidence or can a tendency to appendicitis be inherited?

A Yes, it is possible that you have an inherited tendency. It may be that you have all inherited a similarly shaped appendix. One that is long and thin will block more easily than one that is short and stubby, and so cause appendicitis.

Q I am 45 and have heard that it is highly unlikely that I will ever have appendicitis at my age. Is this true?

A Yes, it is. If you have reached middle life without having had appendicitis, the chances are that you are unlikely to get it now because the appendix shrivels as you get older and is completely shrivelled by the age of 45—so it is not likely to become irritated and inflamed. This is why appendicitis tends to be a complaint of young people.

Q I have heard that swallowing cherry stones can lead to appendicitis. As they are my favourite fruit, I am worried that I may get this problem. Is there any truth in this?

A When appendectomies were first performed years ago, surgeons thought that the small hard lumps they found in the appendix were cherry stones because they looked like them, but in fact they were fecoliths—that is, small lumps of feces which had become trapped in the appendix because it leads nowhere. So you can continue eating your favourite fruit because swallowing fruit stones usually results in their being excreted from the body in the normal way and only very rarely will they cause any irritation to the appendix.

the umbilicus to the top of the pelvic bone. This is called McBurney's point, after the American surgeon who first noted it. But the pain can move to the upper abdomen or down in the pelvis. In a woman, this is particularly confusing as it can be mimicked by gynaecological pains from the ovaries or womb. A rectal examination by the doctor may be needed to establish whether this pain is, in fact, caused by an inflamed, tender appendix.

The inflamed appendix often lies on the right leg muscle where it joins the back. Because this makes the leg stiff, the patient naturally bends the leg up to gain relief. Stretching it down then produces pain. The muscles in the front wall of the abdomen also go into spasm to protect the appendix from any painful movements the patient may make.

It may also be difficult, initially, for the doctor to diagnose appendicitis in children. The child may have a chest infection, with symptoms that imitate appendicitis, which disappear as the respiratory infection improves. But the appendicitis may be genuine, brought on by this other infection swelling the child's glands.

So even if a child seems to have obvious signs of chest trouble, it is very important to tell the doctor if he or she also has a tummyache.

When to see the doctor

If the pain has continued for a whole day or night and has become increasingly severe, and if the patient is vomiting and unable to get up, then it is clearly time to seek medical help. It may be quicker to take the patient to the doctor's surgery, rather than wait for him to call. Home treatments, such as painkillers or soothing drinks should not be tried at this stage. An operation may be urgently needed, and the stomach must be empty of food and drink before an anaesthetic can be given.

Dangers of appendicitis

If the problem is neglected, the situation can become dangerous. The tip of the appendix can become gangrenous, causing perforation. If pus spreads into the abdominal cavity, the result can be a serious inflammation—called peritonitis —which can happen within hours. This can be localized in adults, but in children under 10, it can turn into general peritonitis. When the appendix is removed, a plastic drain has to be inserted to allow any infected matter to drain away. Intravenous fluids (a drip) and antibiotics will also be given to combat the infection and speed the child's recovery.

Appendectomy

Because the risks of neglecting appendi-

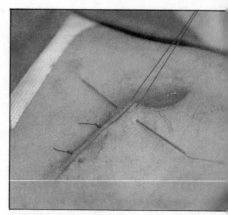

After an appendectomy the wound is carefully stitched so that only the smalles scar will remain.

citis are greater than the risks of an u necessary operation, the surgeon wi operate, even if in doubt. But, if the sym toms are inconclusive, the patient may I put to bed and kept under observation. things do not improve, an operation wi be performed.

The operation is quite simple and on takes about half an hour, under gener anaesthetic. Modern drugs and antibi tics have greatly reduced the risk of cor plications. When the appendix has gon the patient feels much better and is read to leave hospital a few days later. Th stitches at the site of the operation a removed after a week.

The healing process

Once the stitches have been taken ou the scar still has to heal but the patie can soon lead a reasonably normal li again, though active sports, like footba or boxing are out of the question fo several weeks.

After-effects

Occasional twinges of pain will be fe during the healing stage, but these wi disappear within a month or so. Howeve the patient may develop severe wind short time after the operation. Thi happens because the abdomen has bee opened during surgery and air can ente the intestine when the appendix i removed.

Also, after any abdominal operation the bowels cease working and so passin wind is a good sign because it shows tha the digestive system is resuming it normal function—and this means tha the patient can eat and drink again. So patients feel any embarrassment, th best possible reassurance you can give to point out that passing wind is a sig that their body is just getting back t normal and that they are well on the wa to complete recovery.

Appetite

If appetite and hunger were the same no one would be overweight or too thin—we would all eat the right amount to satisfy hunger and nourish ourselves. So what causes appetite and what is its purpose?

When you want to eat something because it looks good, smells nice and tastes delicious, your appetite is working. But when you want to eat something because your stomach is rumbling and you feel in need of food, then your hunger drive is working. This is the basic difference between appetite and hunger.

It is quite an important difference because it is not hunger that makes you overeat, but appetite. In the same way, although you might actually be hungry and need food, your appetite can stop you eating and so the body's needs are not satisfied. This happens in some diseases and in a condition such as anorexia nervosa, where the person becomes obsessed with dieting.

So, it seems that the body's way of letting us know our food requirements is via hunger. Also, it seems that appetite sometimes interferes, not letting the body get the right amount of nourishment. In this case, why do we have appetite, where does it come from, and are there times when it has a really useful role to play?

Developing an appetite

When a baby is born, one of the very first things he or she feels is the need for food. In most cases, this need is satisfied with milk, either from the mother's breast or from a bottle. At this stage in the baby's life, he or she shows no real preference for any type of food. The baby will cry when hungry and be calm and smiling when fed. It is only later that babies will learn what foods they really like.

With this learning, the growing child's appetites are gradually developed. It is because human beings are so complex that we have such different appetites and likes for different foods.

It is interesting to note that in countries that do not share our normal diet, things that we consider to be absolutely inedible are thought to be delicious delicacies. It is also quite revealing that in countries where there is starvation, people do not get the chance to exercise their appetites and are hungry enough to eat virtually anything to keep themselves alive.

How appetite works

Appetite is the regulator of our daily food intake, and thus the eventual regulator of how much we weigh. Because of this, many scientists are very interested in precisely what controls the appetite and they have found that it is quite a complicated process.

In most people, when the appetite is satisfied, eating stops. It is what causes this that is so interesting. It might seem obvious that when you are full you stop eating, but experiments have shown that it is not just a full stomach that tells the brain to stop. For instance, it has been found that there is a hormone produced by the intestines that signals the brain to stop eating.

Other signals come from the concentration of nutrients in the blood, the

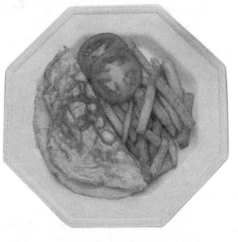

Colour and presentation have much to do with stimulating appetite. This food is nutritionally balanced and attractive.

The same food coloured blue (the most unappetizing colour) and green is not likely to stimulate anyone's appetite.

Di Lewis

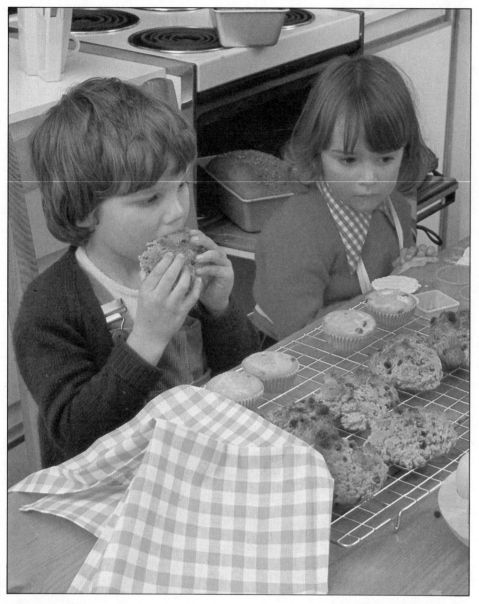

Di Lewis

The aroma of warm, freshly-baked bread and buns is sure to encourage children's appetites, particularly if they have helped to make them.

amount of food that has passed through the mouth and the degree of fullness of the stomach. All these signals are picked up by an area of the brain called the hypothalamus.

Scientists have discovered that there are two separate areas in the hypothalamus that are in charge of eating. One of them controls eating and the other controls satiety, or satisfaction of appetite. The name given to these two areas together is the appestat.

So, all these signals go to the appestat and when there are enough from the areas that are concerned with eating, the appestat tells the brain that the body has had enough and eating stops. This all

sounds very simple, but, unfortunately, it does not always work quite like this. If it did, no one would be overweight or too thin, but this is obviously not the case. So what happens?

Fat and thin

One theory for this is that fat people, or those that eat more than they need, have an appestat that is set too high. In other words, the appestat does not tell the brain to stop eating soon enough.

The opposite is true for thin people: they stop eating too soon. But this theory does not take into account any of the other reasons for over or underweight.

It has been found that fat people are more likely to eat when they see food in front of them, while a person with normal weight will only eat when hungry. Also, fat people pay more attention to the taste of food.

A normal weight person seems to ca less about the food than the fact that he she is taking in fuel to keep the bo running. So, at mealtimes fat people w eat out of habit and eat more than th need, if the food tastes good, and norm weight people will eat only enough satisfy their hunger, without real caring too much about what the fo actually tastes like.

But, again, this does not take account things like eating binges that all peop who are overweight know about only t well. Also, people eat for a number reasons that have nothing to do with fo taste or the regularity of mealtimes. A of theories put forward say that peop eat to compensate for some frustration because they are bored and lone Everyone who has raided the fridge in t middle of the night will know that th are really doing it because they want gain some sort of emotional satisfacti and comfort from the act of eating—a not to relieve any need for food.

Abnormal appetite

There are times in almost everyone' life when, for one reason or another, a abnormal appetite develops. This can b a time when less is eaten, more is eate or even very unusual foods are eaten.

During illness, it is quite common fo people to go off their food. At th moment there is no rational explanatio as to why this happens, as often it i very much in the sick person's interest to eat properly. Doctors think that ther might be subtle changes in the work ings of the body that simply reduce bot hunger and appetite.

Another common type of unusua appetite can happen during pregnancy The stories of pregnant mothers eating all sorts of strange foods or combinatio of foods are legion. There is even likelihood that the hormone changes ir early pregnancy actually change th sense of taste, making previously pleasant foods or drinks taste strange and unpalatable. The eating of very un usual things like coal and earth does no seem to be so common these days, anc doctors think that this behaviour wa caused by the mother needing to make up a mineral deficiency. In this case, the body appears to be cleverer than a lot o people think, as it can tell what unusua food to eat—to make up a deficiency— without the person knowing why.

Generally speaking, fads during preg nancy need not be a cause of anxiety But a sick person who does not want tc eat should be tempted with interesting dishes to take nourishment.

Arteries and artery disease

Q **I have been told that smoking causes artery disease. Is this true?**

A Yes. Hardening of the arteries (arteriosclerosis) is aggravated by smoking, although exactly how this happens is unclear. But there is no doubt that nicotine in the bloodstream does cause arteries to narrow. After a while, they become permanently rigid and less able to carry blood to all parts of the body, particularly the heart—resulting in heart attacks—and the extremities (hands and feet). If blood cannot reach the extremities, tissues degenerate, gangrene sets in, and a limb may have to be amputated.

However, if smoking is given up in time, damage can be avoided.

Q **I jog regularly. Will this reduce the chance of my having a heart attack?**

A There is a reasonable amount of evidence to suggest that regular exercise does have a protective effect against heart attacks, but this is by no means conclusive. A recent study comparing the chances of heart attacks among bus drivers with bus conductors showed a small difference in favour of the conductors, whose job is more active than the drivers'. So it seems reasonable to assume that exercise is a preventive measure and jogging a good idea.

Q **Three of my male relatives, including my father, have died of heart attacks. Are men more prone to atheriosclerosis than women?**

A This does appear to be so, for several reasons. Firstly, female hormones seem to protect women from atheroma (the build-up of fatty deposits in the arteries, which can cause blockages); after the menopause, with its fall in the level of hormone production, atheroma increases. Secondly, until recently, more men smoked than women, but now the pattern is altering and, as a result, the number of women suffering from atheroma before and after the menopause is rising. The conclusion is obvious: give up smoking.

The arteries carry blood containing nourishment and oxygen to all parts of the body. Artery disease is therefore very dangerous, so preventive measures are essential and early treatment vital.

The arteries and veins are the two sorts of large blood vessels in the body. The arteries are like pipes, carrying blood outwards from the heart to the tissues while the veins carry the blood on the return journey. The entire body depends on blood for its supply of oxygen and other vital substances without which life could not go on indefinitely.

The artery network

The heart is a pump which propels blood around the body through the arteries. The main pumping chamber on the left side of the heart, which is called the left ventricle, ejects blood into the main artery of the body – the aorta. The aorta is a tube about 2.5 cm across on the inside.

The first of its branches arise from

The arterial system

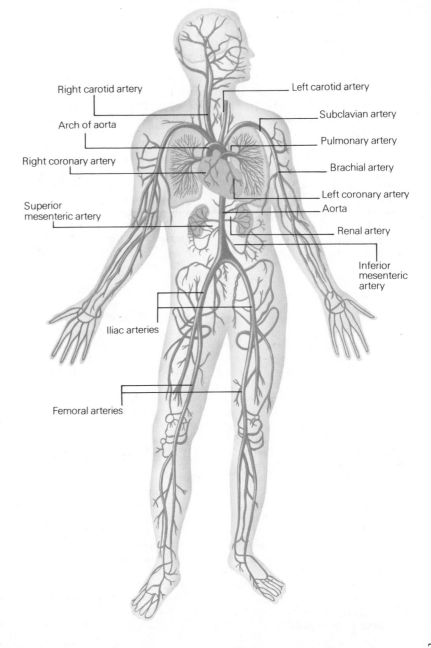

Right carotid artery

Arch of aorta

Right coronary artery

Superior mesenteric artery

Iliac arteries

Femoral arteries

Left carotid artery

Subclavian artery

Pulmonary artery

Brachial artery

Left coronary artery

Aorta

Renal artery

Inferior mesenteric artery

Venner Artists

Development of atherosclerosis

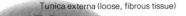

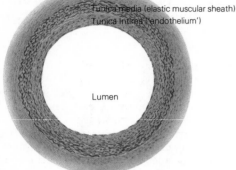

Tunica externa (loose, fibrous tissue)
Tunica media (elastic muscular sheath)
Tunica Intima ('endothelium')

Lumen

Mike Courteney

Fatty streaks
(atherosclerotic lesions)

Lumen

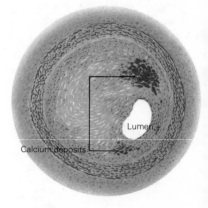

Lumen

Calcium deposits

The normal artery is thick-walled and consists of three layers surrounding the lumen, through which the blood flows.

In a moderate case of atherosclerosis, fatty deposits begin to be built up in the inner layer of the artery.

Here, atherosclerosis is almost total: fatty deposits have severely decreased the lumen and calcium is forming.

the aorta as soon as it leaves the heart. These are the coronary arteries which supply blood to the heart itself. The coronary arteries are particularly likely arteries to be affected by disease. A blocked coronary artery—or coronary thrombosis—causes a heart attack.

After giving rise to the coronary arteries, the aorta passes upward before doubling back on itself in an arch. Originating from this arch are the two main arteries to the head, the left and right carotid arteries, and one artery to each arm. The aorta descends down the chest and into the abdomen.

In the abdomen there are three main arteries to the intestines and the liver, and one to each kidney before the aorta divides into the left and right iliac arteries which supply blood to the pelvis and the legs.

After passing through the capillaries—a network of tiny blood vessels linking the smallest arteries and veins—from which oxygen and nourishment enter the tissues, the blood returns towards the heart in the veins. In general, the artery and vein supplying an area tend to run side by side. The veins empty into the right side of the heart, from where blood is pumped to the lungs and recharged with oxygen. From the lungs, oxygen-rich blood is drained by the pulmonary veins into the left side of the heart.

Here, it starts off round the body again by being pumped into the aorta by the left ventricle of the heart. The left ventricle generates a considerable pressure to force the blood through the arterial network. The tightness which the inflatable cuff used in taking blood-pressure around your arm reaches is the same as the maximum squeeze in the left ventricle with each heartbeat.

The structure of arteries

Since the arteries are subjected to this force with each heartbeat, they have to be thick-walled to cope with the pressure. The outer wall of an artery is a loose, fibrous tissue sheath. Inside this there is a thick, elastic and muscular sheath which gives the artery its strength. There are also rings of muscle fibres encircling the artery in among the elastic tissue. The inner layer of the artery is made of a smooth layer of cells which allows the blood to flow freely (the endothelium).

The thick elastic walls are most important to the system. Much of the force of each heartbeat is taken up in the elastic walls of the big arteries. They continue to push the blood forward in the pause between each heartbeat.

Artery disease

Arterial disease in any part of the body is dangerous because if an artery is blocked or narrowed it is possible that the part it supplies will die from oxygen starvation. There are two basic ways in which a blockage can happen.

Hardening of the arteries is the commonest serious illness in the Western world. Age is the most important cause, but many other factors affect the rate at which arterial disease progresses.

The changes in the walls of arteries which lead to hardening are called arteriosclerosis ('sclerosis' means hardening). These changes are caused by the development of an excessive amount of fibrous tissue. This can happen as a result of straining of the artery walls caused by raised blood pressure.

The other type of disease is atheroma, which is the name given to fatty deposits which attach themselves to the arterial

walls increasingly with advancing ag These fatty deposits look like porrid and 'atheroma' is Greek for porridge.

Changes in the arterial netwo resulting from atheroma, as opposed arteriosclerosis are usually referred to atherosclerosis—a word your doctor more likely to use than arteriosclero Arterio—and atherosclerosis are wor which can be used interchangeably.

Cholesterol

The atheromatous process first sta with a deposit of cholesterol—a norm constituent of the blood and one the building blocks of normal cells— the wall of the artery. However, it see that cholesterol leaks into the inn surface (intima) of the artery and a 'fa streak' forms within the arterial wall.

As the fatty streak grows in size a depth two other things happen. First, t surface of the streak may break down a expose the middle portions of the arter wall to the blood. When this happens triggers the mechanism for clotting t blood. A clot normally forms as a plug fibrous tissue to stop bleeding from wound. When the process occurs aroun fatty streak, a mixture of fibrous a fatty tissue is formed in the arterial w and this is called an atheromato plaque. As the plaque grows it starts encroach upon the central blood-fill space—that is, the lumen of the artery.

Finally, the development of the plaq involves changes occurring deep in t arterial wall. Fibrous tissue forms on t inner surface of the original fatty strea but there is also a growth of fibrous tiss on the wall side of the plaque, growi from the outside of the artery towards centre. The end result is a mixture fibrous and fatty tissue blocking proportion of the arterial lumen. T

...sease extends to a considerable depth in ...e wall of the vessel and encroaches on a ...rge proportion of its circumference.

Once a large atheromatous plaque has ...rmed it may have a number of con- ...quences. It may steadily enlarge to ...ock the artery. Because the artery is ...rtially blocked, the flow of blood past ...e obstruction is reduced. This may ...tivate the clotting system at the site of ...rrowing. The clot may well produce a ...mplete obstruction known as a ...rombosis. Atheromatous plaques ...hich are partly blocking an artery may ...come displaced and swing across the ...men of the artery, like a lock gate, to ...ock it completely. Parts of an athero- ...atous plaque may break off and travel ...wards a smaller artery which will then ...come blocked. This is a phenomenon ...nown as embolism.

Atheroma can affect any artery ...wn to a diameter of about 2 milli- ...etres. However, the process is most ...kely to occur in areas of arterial wall ...hich are subjected to movement and ...ost stress. For this reason, atheroma is ...mmonest at sites where arteries branch ...to smaller arteries. There is a greater ...retching of the lining of the arteries at ...ese points allowing more cholesterol to ...t into the wall.

...he results of blockage

...nce arteries are necessary to supply ...xygen to every part of the body, there is ...o organ which is completely immune to ...e effects of arterial disease. If an organ ...a limb has its blood supply cut off by ...heroma then it must eventually die. An ...ea of tissue which has lost its oxygen ...pply is called an area of infarction. ...hen this process occurs in an arm or a ...g it is more usual to use the term ...ngrene.

There are obviously some areas where ...e effects of atheroma cause especially ...vere problems. The most important are ...e heart, the brain, the legs and, finally, ...e aorta itself.

...eart attacks

...theroma particularly affects the heart ...cause the two coronary arteries, the ...teries that supply blood to the heart, ...e under more mechanical stress than ...actically any other arteries in the body. ...he heart is continuously contracting ...d relaxing with each heartbeat and, in ...doing, the coronary arteries, which lie ...the outer surface of the heart, are ...ternately stretched and relaxed. This ...ems to give ideal conditions for ...heromatous plaques to be formed. ...hen a coronary artery becomes blocked ...s a result of atheroma, then a heart ...tack results. Such an event may also be

known as a coronary thrombosis, or a myocardial infarction (the 'myocardium' is the heart muscle and infarction is the formation of a dead area of the muscle when it is deprived of blood).

But heart attacks are not the only problem which atheroma causes in the heart. Where there is a fixed obstruction which is not totally blocking the artery, the supply of blood to the heart may only be sufficient to meet the needs of the body when at rest. Exercise increases the need for blood in the heart and it becomes starved of oxygen. This causes pain arising in the heart which is known as angina pectoris, or simply angina. The two problems of angina and myocardial infarction are often lumped together under the title of ischaemic heart disease, ischaemia being a word which implies a lack of oxygen without total deprivation or infarction.

Strokes

In the brain atherosclerosis may result in a stroke. These may vary from the trivial to the fatal and may occur as a result of an artery becoming blocked through atheroma or embolism or through an artery leaking blood into the brain as a result of a weakened wall.

When the legs are severely affected by atheroma they become painful and this pain is worse during exercise, just as with angina. If the disease is severe, then gangrene results and the affected leg may have to be amputated.

Finally, the aorta itself is a very important area of atheromatous disease. Two different things can happen. The

An arteriogram is an X-ray in which dye is injected into the bloodstream to detect blockages. This arteriogram of an upper leg is normal and shows no blockage.

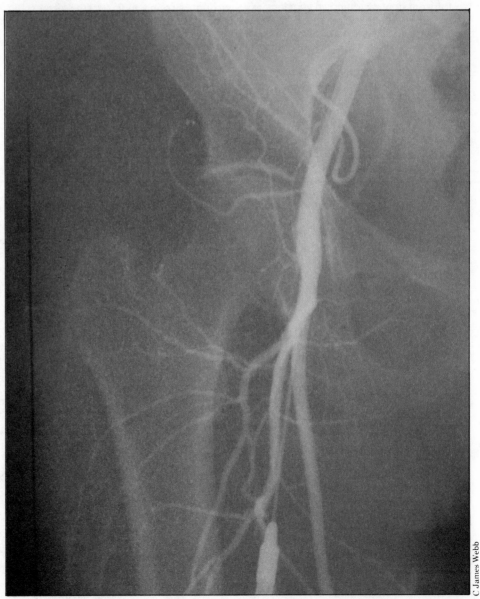

C James Webb

Q I know that smoking is bad for me. But will alcohol also increase the likelihood of my getting a bad heart?

A There is no evidence that moderate amounts of alcohol make atheroma worse; indeed, there are pointers in the opposite direction. Moderation, however, should still be observed. An excess is harmful in other ways.

Q I have arterial disease. Should I try and keep my legs warm?

A If you are suffering from peripheral vascular disease which reduces — and can prevent — blood flow to the extremities, you may be feeling the cold. Unfortunately, warming up your legs will only increase their demand for oxygen which is supplied by the blood. In hospital, legs badly afflicted by arterial disease are deliberately kept cool in the hope of preserving them. I should take further advice from your own doctor who knows the history of your condition.

Q My husband and I eat a lot of of meat and dairy products. Do you think I should cut my husband's intake down, as I am worried about its cholestrol content?

A There are several very important points here. Firstly, if your husband smokes, there is no point in doing anything until he stops, as this will counteract the good effects of any other measures.

Secondly, you should be aware that there is more to a prudent diet than simply cutting down on cholesterol intake. Most of this comes from the body's own chemical processes anyway, and it is these that the prudent diet should aim to alter. It would seem sensible to move the diet towards more unrefined carbohydrate — that is, foods containing a lot of roughage like wholemeal bread and bran.

Then try and reduce all fats, in particular animal fats and dairy produce — called 'saturated fats', replacing them with those of vegetable origin. A diet such as this will reduce the intake of cholesterol while at the same time having a dramatic effect on the cholesterol already in the blood.

wall of the aorta may start to balloon out as a result of the weakening effect of the disease. This produces sack-like swelling called an aneurism instead of the regular tubular structure of the normal aorta. Aneurisms are usually found in the abdomen but may occur in the chest. An aneurism may continue to expand and eventually start to leak, with disastrous results. Surgical treatment is the only hope and it is necessary to strengthen the aorta with a woven fabric tube. The results of this sort of surgery when carried out as an emergency are often good, although there are failures.

Another form of aneurism which tends to occur in the chest rather than the abdomen, is called dissection of the aorta. This means that the layers of the aortic wall become split by escaping blood, the end result being much the same. Occasionally, patients survive dissection without surgery but, again, surgery is usually necessary.

Those affected

There is now a well-established list of risk factors which indicate people who are more likely to suffer from 'accelerated' or 'early' atheroma. For instance, some diseases put people at greater risk. The two most important are high blood pressure and diabetes.

People from a family in which athero- clerosis has occurred are at greater risk developing problems themselves. An finally, there is the cholesterol level the blood. Although this is a definite ri factor, the value of cholester measurements in individuals h perhaps been overemphasized. Howeve it does seem sensible to reduce th amount of meat and dairy products your diet.

Prevention

What can we do to prevent or postpone th development of atheromatous diseas Obviously both diabetes and high bloc pressure must be treated. If there are predisposing illnesses, then the mo potent risk factor is family history, ov which there is no control. However, the is one controllable factor left — smokin The most effective thing to preve atheroma is to stop smoking, for it ca counteract the benefits of oth measures. Apart from significant reducing the chances of your developi heart disease, giving up cigarettes wi generally improve your health.

This thermograph, or heat-sensitive picture, shows the effects of smoking o the circulation. Note the decreased blood flow to the fingertips.

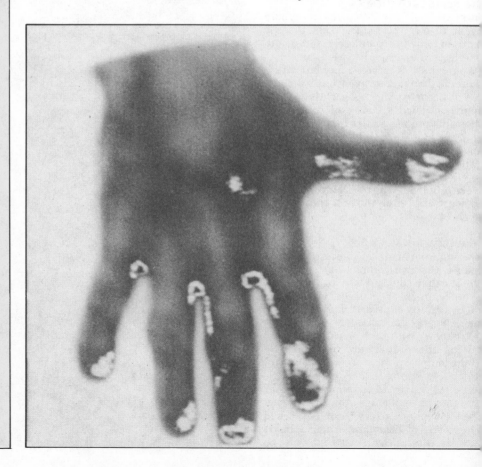

Arthritis

Q An old countryman once told me that he avoided arthritis by keeping a piece of cut potato in his pocket. Is there anything in this?

A You might as well believe that the moon is made of green cheese! Although many herbs have proven medicinal properties, the potato is not one of them. Your friend was just lucky enough not to have developed arthritis.

Q Is it safe to take a lot of aspirin to ease pain caused by arthritis?

A Yes and no. Because aspirin reduces inflammation and temperature and eases pain, it is often used as a first-line treatment for arthritis. Unfortunately, there are two side-effects that can happen when aspirin is taken for a long time. Bleeding can start from tiny gastric ulcers or an existing ulcer can flare up. If you start vomiting blood, or something that looks like coffee grounds, or pass black, tar-like bowel motions—stop taking the aspirin and seek medical help. The risk of stomach upsets is greatly reduced if you always use soluble aspirin. Another side effect is ringing in the ears—if this happens, reduce the amount of aspirin.

Q Are some occupations more likely to cause arthritis than others?

A Regrettably, yes. Doctors are familiar with various 'wear and tear' effects, such as 'baker's cyst'—which is fluid at the back of the knee produced by excessive bending (when getting bread in and out of the oven), 'porter's neck'—which is osteoarthritis of the neck joints, caused by tilting the neck (when carrying objects over the shoulder), and even 'ballet dancer's toe'—which looks like a bunion.

Q Can I do any good to an inflamed joint if I rub liniment on it?

A Very little, but you may find it soothing. Vegetable oil or soap liniment are cheapest and as good as anything. For a bruised joint, massage with emollients may help.

Many people are affected by some form of arthritis, which can range from temporary discomfort to a more serious disability, but medical help and physiotherapy can do much to relieve the condition.

Arthritis is an inflammation of the joints and its causes are as varied and mysterious as the condition itself. It affects people of all ages and is a common complaint in temperate climates; it can be mild or severe, affecting one joint or several; and the different types include rheumatoid arthritis, osteoarthritis, rigid spine disease (*ankylosing spondylitis*) and arthritis that has been brought on by an injury or other infection. Although its study is a well-established speciality, called rheumatology, medical research cannot yet tell us all the answers.

Rheumatoid arthritis in adults
Although it is common, the cause of rheumatoid arthritis is unknown. It is thought that it may be due to an 'auto-immune' phenomenon—that is, some event, perhaps a severe illness or a shock which triggers a chain of chemical reactions within the body eventually producing chemicals which react against the body's own tissues—in this case, against the lining tissue of the joints—the

This X-ray shows a badly diseased arthritic hip. Suitable treatment would be hip joint replacement.

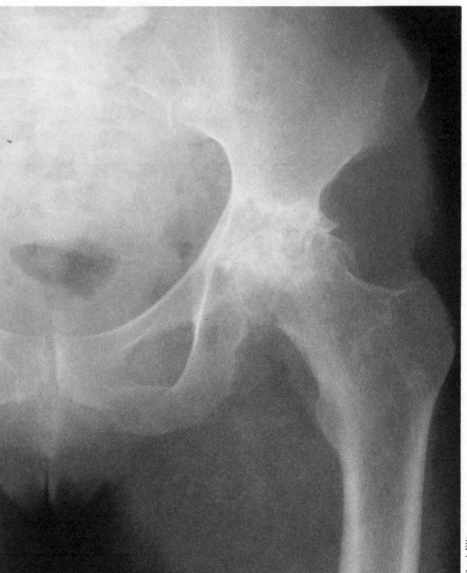

synovium. Inflammation and arthritis will follow.

Rheumatoid arthritis usually affects adults between the ages of 20 and 55, and women are three times more liable to it than men. Inflammation of the knuckles of both hands is the usual symptom, and the joints of the toes are affected in a similar way. At the same time, the sufferer may lose weight, feel unwell and become lethargic. The symptoms may be either acute, starting with a fever or rash, or happen gradually over several weeks.

The joints most often affected are the knees, hips, shoulders, wrists, elbows, ankles and the bones of the neck. The stiffness is usually at its worst in the mornings, and in acute cases the sufferer may be confined to bed or have great difficulty with movement.

In about one quarter of cases, attacks will last about six months, but only happen every few years. Some cases are persistent, varying in severity, but tending to 'burn out' after many years.

In children
Rheumatoid arthritis can occur in children—a condition called Still's disease—but it is fortunately rare. Two main age groups are affected—between one and three and 10 and 15. The inflammation starts gradually, and in about one third of cases occurs in one joint

only, commonly the knee. It can also affect the hands, wrists, feet and ankles.

This disease is slowly progressive, but burns itself out in late adolescence. The chances of a cure depend on the severity of the case, how early it is diagnosed and how quickly treatment is begun. It should be started early to prevent permanent stiffening and joint deformity .

Osteoarthritis
Osteoarthritis occurs as part of the ageing process. It happens mainly to weight-bearing joints: hips, knees and spine. In women the hands are also often affected, particularly the top joints of the fingers and the base of the thumb.

This condition is caused by a degeneration of the cartilage, a tough, elastic tissue which protects the surface of the joint. This is normally glistening and smooth, but osteoarthritis causes it to roughen and the cartilage becomes 'dry'. This change has two effects: it compresses the underlying bone surface that the cartilage should protect and inflames the synovium (the lining) lying over it.

The first symptoms are pain and loss of use; stiffness and swelling follow, and the joint eventually changes shape. There may be only one joint involved, such as the right hip in a right-handed person (because right-handedness means that the right side of the body is more active

and bears more weight then the left), o in many cases, the knees, spir shoulders, hands and neck are affecte This condition is also slowly progressiv but disability rarely happens unless t arthritis in a weight-bearing joint severe. Unfortunately, any injury w cause the condition to flare up.

Rigid spine disease
Ankylosing spondylitis is a form arthritis which affects the pelvic join and spine. This, too, is thought to be auto-immune illness, like rheumato arthritis, but there is a definite tenden for it to run in families. It is more comm in men, usually starting between the ag of 15 and 30.

The inflammation causes calcium to deposited in the ligaments (fibrous ban which connect joints). This results stiffness which can lead to the spin bones (the vertebrae) being fus together if the inflammation is n alleviated by both medical treatment ar exercise—hence its colloquial nam 'poker back'. The illness progress slowly for a few years, often spreading the whole spine and involving the h joints, before gradually petering out.

Other causes of arthritis
An injury can trigger arthritis—this called 'traumatic' arthritis. The inju

Comparison of a normal and an osteoarthritic knee joint

In osteoarthritis some cartilage, which lines the bones of the knee joint, forms into lumps (osteophytes) and some wears away. As it wears, bones lose thei protection which causes pain.

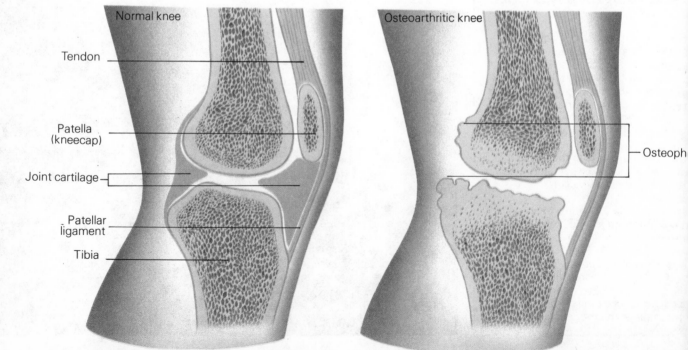

Normal knee

Tendon

Patella (kneecap)

Joint cartilage

Patellar ligament

Tibia

Osteoarthritic knee

Osteoph

Types of arthritis and their treatment

Type	Cause	Symptoms	Treatment
Rheumatoid arthritis	'Auto immune', i.e. chain of reactions in body	Lethargy, high temperature, rash (occasionally)	Anti-inflammatory drugs, painkilling drugs, gold injections or steroid drugs. Immediate hospital treatment for children. Reducing swelling by drawing off (aspirating) fluid, physiotherapy, exercise, splinting, joint replacement
	Affects adults between 20 & 55 also children (Still's disease)	Pain, swelling, redness, stiffness and loss of function in joints of fingers or toes.	
Osteoarthritis	Wear and tear due to ageing; degeneration of cartilage over joint	Pain, followed by stiffness, swelling, change of shape	Basic principles as above
Ankylosing spondylitis	'Auto immune' – possibly hereditary, more common in males between 15 & 30, calcium deposited in joint ligaments	Stiff lower back in mornings, pain on bending spine	Anti-inflammatory drugs, exercise
Traumatic	Injury e.g. falling heavily	Joint becomes inflamed, painful and swollen a few hours after injury	Rest, bandaging, painkilling drugs, then physiotherapy. X-ray in case of fracture, possible aspiration of fluid

...n either be direct, for example from a ...low to a joint, or indirect, as when you ...urt your knee by falling heavily on it. ...raumatic arthritis usually happens to ...en, although no-one is immune.

The knee, ankle or wrist are the joints ...ost-commonly affected. A few hours ...fter the injury, the joint becomes ...flamed, painful and swollen. An X-ray ... needed, in case a fracture has occurred, ...ut rest, bandaging and painkillers may ... all that is necessary.

Physiotherapy can also help restore ...obility and muscle power to the affected ...mb. Occasionally the injury causes ...eeding into the joint which becomes ...ery tense and painful; this may have to ... drawn out with a needle (aspirated) ...nder a local anaesthetic.

Germs can also cause conditions like ...eptic arthritis, which is brought on by a ...erm in the joint fluid. This happens ...ther because of an injury or because it is ...ansmitted from the blood. Half of such ...ses involve the knee, but it can occur in ...ny large joint. Both children and the ...derly can be affected, but it is ...rtunately rare.

Another rare form of arthritis can ...esult from an attack of German measles ...ubella). This can happen to adults, who ...ay experience swelling of their finger ...ints, knees and ankles which subsides ...fter a few weeks.

Arthritis of the lower spine and hip, ...esulting from tuberculosis, is now also ...are except in people from the developing ...ountries. Other infections such as ...eumatic fever, gonorrhoea and the skin ...sease psoriasis, can also give rise to ...rthritis.

...iagnosis and treatment

...you suspect that you have some form of ...rthritis, the worst thing you can do is to 'just put up with it'. Do not try to make the diagnosis yourself, but go and see your doctor. Any delay might mean the risk of permanent deformity, especially in the case of a child with Still's disease, a condition which needs hospital care.

Your doctor will ask for a history of your illness and give you an examination. He may prescribe drugs such as aspirin, indomethacin and ibuprofen, which combat inflammation and ease pain, and painkillers like acetaminophen or distalgesic tablets, which are stronger. Gold injections may be given in the affected joints, but these can have unpleasant side-effects and are used only when absolutely necessary.

You may have to rest the affected joints or wear an individually-made splint to keep them in the best position and so prevent deformities from occurring. Swelling in joints can be treated by

Coping with arthritis at home

- Build ramp to replace outdoor steps.
- Make door openings wide enough to take wheelchair, if necessary.
- Fix handrail on both sides of stairs
- Replace worn carpets; keep floor space clear for walking aids.
- Raise electric sockets about 1m (3 ft) above ground.
- Replace light switches with pull cords.
- Fix wire basket inside door below letter box to save bending.
- Raise heights of chairs with blocks fixed to ends of chair legs; raise height of seat with firm cushions.
- To increase leverage on refrigerator handle, slip loop of leather, or strong string over handle.
- Pad handles of utensils (e.g. potato peeler) with foam rubber; also brush and broom handles.
- Use basket on wheels to carry things from one room to another.
- Fix handrails to bath and around toilet; raised toilet seat.
- Iron and ironing board fixed to wall to avoid carrying.
- Electric ripple' bed-current ripples through plastic mattress to give cushioning effect.
- Long-handled garden tools.
- Adjustable seat in bath.
- Lightweight carpet sweeper.
- Extend toilet seat for wheelchair users.
- Washing machine and kitchen surfaces at convenient heights.

Q **My doctor says I have a 'frozen shoulder'. Is that a form of arthritis?**

A No. It is simply a condition that mimics it. Others in this category include 'tennis elbow' and nerve-pain in the wrist, which is called carpal tunnel syndrome. What these conditions have in common is inflammation of the tissues around a joint—but in each case, other evidence confirming arthritis is absent.

Q **My daughter is severely affected by arthritis but she is planning to get married in the very near future. What are her chances of enjoying any sex life or starting a family?**

A When either partner has arthritis, they will want answers to many questions before they start a family. An important point is whether their children will be especially prone to this condition. Only one type of arthritis, caused by haemophilia is clearly inherited. With many other forms the chances of an affected parent handing on the disease are rare. In an acute phase of the disease, it would be painful to attempt sex, but otherwise it is quite safe to have intercourse.

Q **My grandmother always wears a bandage on her arthritic knee. Is this really helpful?**

A Bandaging or supporting an acutely inflamed joint can stop any jarring movement and therefore ease pain. When a joint is swollen, the tissues feel stretched—a support in these circumstances gives a sensation of stability. Wearing a bandage also serves to warn other people that a knock would *not* be appreciated!

Q **I've been told heat is good for arthritis and am wondering if I could use an infra-red lamp to ease the pain?**

A Heat is soothing and infra-red is a penetrating heat. Place it about 60cm (24in) away from the affected joint and use it for about 20 minutes—up to three times daily. There is no long-term benefit, but it can be useful if done just before you begin an exercise routine.

drawing off excess fluid under a local anaesthetic, or injecting an anti-inflammatory drug into the joint.

You may be feeling generally unwell and be advised to cut down some of your everyday activities and rest as much as possible. Steroid drugs (such as cortisone) may be prescribed to suppress the inflammation in the joints, but because they have side-effects they will only be used when all other forms of treatment have been tried and are unsuccessful. Doses must always be kept at the lowest possible level at which they will carefully control symptoms, and progress must be carefully monitored by a doctor.

If your symptoms persist, your doctor may recommend a visit to the rheumatic clinic of your local hospital for further investigation. An acute attack of arthritis with fever, swollen joints and a general feeling of being unwell may need immediate hospital treatment, including splinting and rest on a special 'ripple' bed—an electric current 'ripples' through a plastic mattress, giving a cushioning effect.

Blood tests are made to establish the type of arthritis involved, to see if you a anaemic, to check the amount inflammation in the body at regul intervals and to assess the progress of t disease. Other tests will show whether t condition is caused by septic arthrit gonococcal (VD) arthritis, or by bleedi into the joint.

Another technique, called arthroscop involves a telescope-type instrume which is used to look inside the knee joi under local anaesthetic. Both t cartilage and lining tissue can examined by this means, and small piec of tissue can be removed for furth microscopic examination to help esta lish the cause of the condition.

Exercise and physiotherapy
Physiotherapy plays an important part the treatment of all forms of arthriti For affected joints that are in a 'quiescer phase—that is, free of inflammatio exercise is essential to prevent stiffne and loss of mobility and restore muscl around the joint that may have waste There is no evidence that exercising a arthritic joint in the quiescent pha

In this adapted kitchen the emphasis is on areas which ensure the maximum of ease and efficiency for arthritics when using their hands or bending.

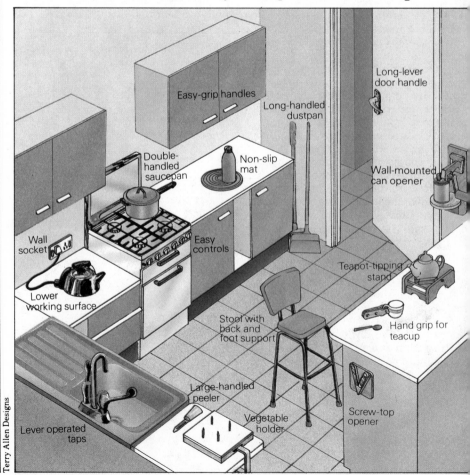

Easy-grip handles

Long-lever door handle

Long-handled dustpan

Double-handled saucepan

Non-slip mat

Wall-mounted can opener

Wall socket

Easy controls

Teapot-tipping stand

Lower working surface

Stool with back and foot support

Hand grip for teacup

Large-handled peeler

Screw-top opener

Vegetable holder

Lever operated taps

Terry Allen Designs

specially important in this bathroom e adaptations that allow the arthritis ffferer to sit comfortably and without

too much bending. Note also the toilet flush which can be pressed and the lever taps in the bathtub.

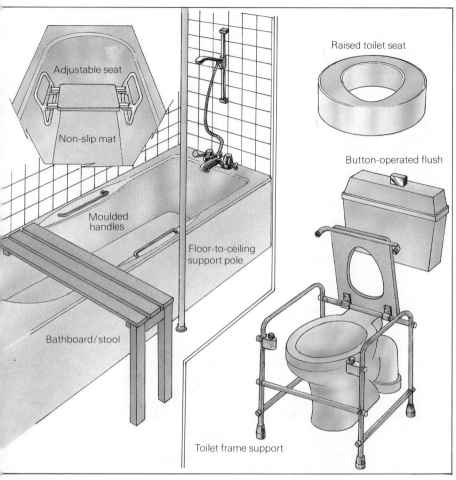

Adjustable seat

Non-slip mat

Moulded handles

Bathboard/stool

Floor-to-ceiling support pole

Raised toilet seat

Button-operated flush

Toilet frame support

there is no cure yet for every disability caused by arthritis, better general care and physical aids can make life more tolerable in many ways.

Aids such as splints, surgical collars, walking sticks and frames, elbow crutches, wheelchairs and some of the more complicated electrical hoisting aids can all be matched to the individual needs by physiotherapists.

Advice can also be obtained from rehabilitation centres about specialized aids to mobility, such as electric wheelchairs.

Replacing one kind of lifestyle with another is always possible, although not always easy. Adjusting your employment must obviously take priority. You may need to change shifts, use specially adapted equipment or generally take on lighter duties. You doctor can help by writing to your employer about your specific problems.

Structural changes in the home may be necessary and there are many helpful adaptations that can be made. Living on one level in a bungalow or apartment is obviously more practical than living in a conventional two-storey house – but where this is not possible the problems caused by steps can be overcome by using special equipment. Nor need hobbies and pastimes as varied as card playing, gardening or needle craft be forgotten. Occupational therapists can advise about the many ingenious devices and techniques that have been developed to enable arthritics to continue enjoying these pleasures.

uses it to flare up.

The physiotherapist at your local spital will teach you exercises which n be continued at home. Heat can be ed to ease painful joints. These treatents can include short-wave diathermy, en a heater pad is placed near the ected joint, or hydrotherapy (exercising a small, very warm swimming pool). e effect of the heat is to relax tense uscles and, because the water supports e weight of the body, movement is creased.

f your doctor or physiotherapist vises it, an infra-lamp can be used at me. Paraffin wax baths for hands and et is another treatment that can be used ry easily at home once the technique is rned. On the other hand, some erapists favour ice packs as a form of in-relieving therapy.

e benefits of surgery

eat advances have been made in the placement of badly-damaged joints th artificial ones. In the first place, the cision that an arthritic joint needs

surgery will be made by a specialist in the field, an orthopaedic surgeon who has been consulted by either the patient's doctor or a rheumatologist. The results of such an operation can be a dramatic relief of pain, correction of deformity and increased movement. The benefits to the patient may include restoring enjoyment of sexual intercourse which may have previously been very difficult.

Surgery can also relieve pressure around a joint, free gummed-up ligaments or remove the inflamed lining tissue of a joint (synovectomy) if it is excessively inflamed. An excruciatingly painful and useless joint such as may occur with osteoarthritis of the cervical spine (neck) or an arthritic knee is sometimes surgically fused (arthrodesis) to give relief, though this does involve loss of movement.

Help available

An active person, who has become seriously disabled, must first come to terms with the feelings of dependence and helplessness that this brings. Although

A physiotherapist helps the victim of arthritis with exercises and techniques such as heat treatment or hydrotherapy.

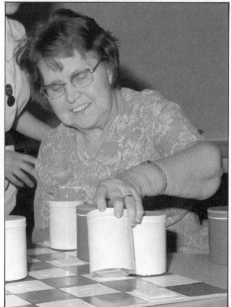

John Watney

Artificial insemination

Q **I have been married for several years and have not become pregnant. After tests on us both, our doctor has suggested artificial insemination, but I am worried that it will affect our marriage.**

A Generally, AIH puts very little strain on a marriage—although some men can feel a sense of failure. However, both you and your husband should realize that he really will be the father of the child and that you can now have the baby you both long for. But if there are already stresses in a marriage, AID should not be undertaken. A husband's disappointment that he cannot be the father of the child, or a wife's resentment at not being able to have a natural child, can be enough to destroy a marriage. So it is very important that any such conflicts are resolved first.

Q **If I have a child by artificial insemination will it be legitimate?**

A A child conceived through AIH is legitimate. The legal position of a child conceived through AID varies from country to country; sometimes a child conceived in this way is not considered legitimate until the parents adopt it.

Q **We have decided to try to have a child by AIH but are worried that it won't work. What is the success rate for artificial insemination?**

A It varies, depending on the fertility of the woman, but, generally speaking, there is a success rate of between 50 and 70 per cent. However, it may be necessary to carry out the treatment for a period of six months to a year before it results in the desired pregnancy.

Q **Is it possible that I will be able to choose the sex of my child if I conceive it by artificial insemination?**

A No. It is no more possible for you to choose the sex of a child you conceive by artificial insemination than it is if you conceive a child during intercourse.

Artificial insemination may seem a radical solution to an infertility problem, but it is in fact a simple medical technique which has enabled many couples to become parents who would otherwise be childless.

The term artificial insemination refers to the process in which sperm is inserted into the female reproductive tract by artificial means rather than through sexual intercourse. The sperm is usually placed next to the woman's cervix (the opening to the womb) using a syringe to which a long tube is attached.

Although increasingly used in cases of infertility, artificial insemination is one of several treatments available when couples fail to conceive. After carrying out tests, a couple's doctor will advise them on whether hormone treatment, surgery or artificial insemination will be the best treatment for them and will explain what is involved.

There are two forms of artificial insemination. If a woman has her husband's sperm inserted into her vagina, the process is called artificial insemination-husband (AIH). However, if the sperm of a different male is inserted, it is called artificial insemination-donor (AID).

Artificial insemination-husband

This method is used when there is some fault with the way the sperm is deposited in the vagina during normal intercourse. It may also be used to overcome some female reproductive problems.

For example, AIH might be used when there is some abnormality in the structure of the penis—a surprising number of men have the opening, whi is usually found at the tip of the pen situated elsewhere along the penile sha Most common of these conditions is whe the opening is on the underside, ba from the tip. So instead of the sperm bei deposited next to the cervix, where th can easily swim up to meet the fema eggs in the fallopian tubes, they a deposited nearer the entrance of t vagina and conception does not ta place. However, by using artifici insemination, the sperm can be plac directly next to the cervix and so increa the chances of conception.

Another case might be when a man unable to achieve an erection or when is unable to ejaculate within the vagir These men may be able to mainta strong erections and have ejaculatio when masturbating, or through manu manipulation by the partner or in or sex, but they lose these abilities as soon penetration is attempted.

For men who have low sperm counts technique called *split ejaculate insemi ation* is used, which also involves AI When the sperm count is low, the numb of sperm in the semen that has be ejaculated may be too low for fertilizati to occur. However, the first part of t ejaculate always contains more sper than the rest and if the first parts several separate ejaculations are p together, then the number of sper

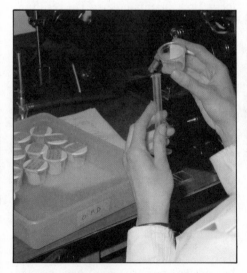

A labelled sample of recently ejaculated sperm is being tested for volume before being classified.

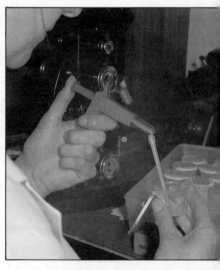

The sample is being diluted with a sali (salt water) solution as a preparation f the taking of a sperm count.

creases. Using AIH, this collection of several ejaculates is introduced into the woman at the time when she is most likely to conceive.

AIH can also be used when the barrier to conception is found in the female partner. For sperm to be able to enter the womb and swim up to fertilize the egg (ovum), they must swim through the right quantity of watery mucus secreted by the cervix: some women produce too little mucus; others produce mucus so thick that the sperm cannot penetrate. AIH may solve this by attempting to put the sperm beyond the barrier.

Most parents tend not to tell the offspring that he or she was conceived through the use of AIH. In fact there is little to be gained by doing so. Besides, most parents usually forget the experience after several years.

Artificial insemination-donor

AID is used when the woman has no reproductive problems but either the man is sterile or the female is allergic to her partner's sperm. In this case, sperm is obtained from an unidentified male and introduced into the female in the same way that it is for AIH.

AID presents a good alternative, allowing a woman to have the experience of carrying and bearing a child which at least inherits *her* characteristics. And, since AID will be used only as a last resort to solve the problem of childlessness, most men feel quite happy about it.

The greatest care is taken in matching the donor's physical characteristics, such as height, build and complexion, with those of the husband, so that the child has the greatest chance of looking like both parents. The donors are also matched for

Artificial insemination by syringe

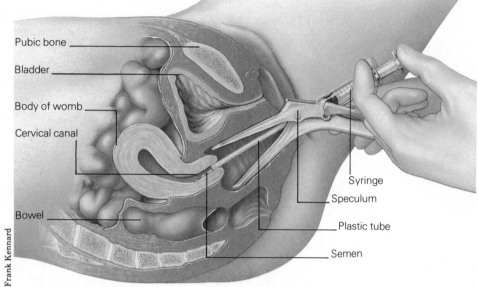

Pubic bone

Bladder

Body of womb

Cervical canal

Bowel

Syringe

Speculum

Plastic tube

Semen

Frank Kennard

intellectual ability.

The donors' medical and family histories are also examined carefully to avoid passing on conditions like diabetes or other inherited ailments. Furthermore, the characteristics of the female partner are also considered. If she does not have the Rh factor in her blood, for example, then a Rh negative donor is used to avoid future complications in pregnancy.

The matching procedures used are so effective that relatives, friends and the child itself do not generally suspect that AID has been used. But, in any case, genetic makeup of the offspring is far less important in the relationship between parents and child than genuine love.

Some doctors mix in some of the

In artificial insemination a warmed speculum (gynecological instrument) opens the vagina while a plastic tube carries the sperm sample from the syringe into the cervical canal.

husband's sperm with that of the donor (except where the woman reacts against her partner's sperm). This provides a small chance that the one sperm to penetrate could, after all, have come from the husband.

Research has shown that the children conceived by artificial insemination show no difference in rates of abnormality than children conceived in any other way.

The treatment
Treatment is carried out at infertility

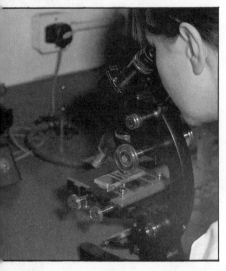

When it has been prepared, the sperm count itself is done under a very high powered microscope.

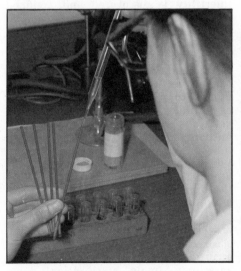

After all the tests have been carried out, the sample is dropped into pipettes (fine glass tubes) just before it is frozen.

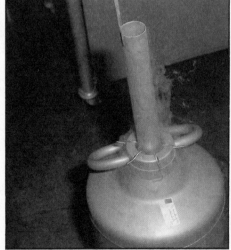

Ken Moreman

Prepared sperm is frozen in low-temperature liquid (liquid nitrogen) inside this sperm bank.

Manfred Kage/Bruce Coleman

clinics attached to gynaecological departments in some of the larger hospitals.

The first session in all cases of infertility consists of an interview with both partners. A medical examination is given to the woman, and a full medical and surgical history is obtained from both the man and the woman. Their attitudes towards one another, towards their infertility and towards children are also carefully discussed.

After this initial joint interview, the couple are usually examined separately: the woman has a gynaecological examination and a swab from her cervix is taken, and the man undergoes a full examination including his genitals.

Over successive sessions at the clinic, the doctors will establish the cause of the infertility. The man will always have to undergo a sperm count to help them do this, which involves giving a fresh specimen of semen. If the man feels he could not 'masturbate to order' at the clinic, he can produce his specimen at home, provided the sample is received at the hospital laboratory within two hours of ejaculation.

Sometimes the man may not be able to ejaculate through masturbating at all. In this case he is encouraged to have intercourse with his partner, but instead of ejaculating into her vagina, he does so into a dry, wide-mouthed jar kept ready by the bed.

The woman will be asked to monitor her basal body temperature–her temperature at rest before she begins any activity–since this provides clues as to

Normal sperm under the microscope (above left) and (above right) magnified 1000 times. A great number of sperms in any ejaculate, however, are abnormal and in many cases will not be able to swim properly: (right, top) this sperm has a head which is too large and a tail that is too short; (centre) this sperm's head is too large and its tail is double; (bottom) this sperm is grossly abnormal.

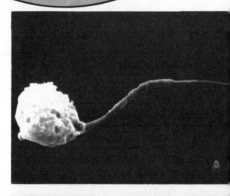

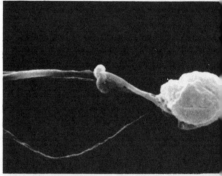

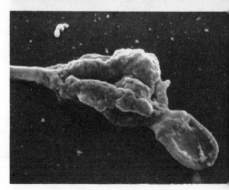

when ovulation is likely to be occurring. This is the time of the month when an egg is released from her ovary and she is at her most fertile. Once the cause of infertility is discovered and artificial insemination considered, the insemination can be arranged to take place at the times of ovulation to increase the chance of conception.

Artificial insemination is generally carried out on three consecutive days around the time of ovulation and may continue for a period of six months to a year. The sperm sample from either the husband or the donor is passed along a tube and inserted into the cervical canal. Where there is a cervical abnormality or a problem with the cervical mucus then the sample may be placed past the cervix within the uterus.

The sperm does not have to be fresh– provided it is frozen quickly following ejaculation, very little deterioration occurs. Indeed many men who undergo vasectomy (male sterilization) have samples of their sperm stored in sperm banks, and these samples have produced healthy children by artificial insemination.

Artificial limbs

Q I recently lost my leg in a car accident and am to be fitted with an artificial limb. I am frightened that it will feel peculiar and painful. Are my fears justified?

A An artificial leg is designed so that its socket fits the 'stump' of the natural limb comfortably. However, weight loss or gain will affect the fit of socket and stump and make the leg less comfortable to wear. If this happens, return to the hospital where the limb was fitted.

The wearing of an artificial limb can sometimes cause sensations of 'phantom pain' and of having a 'phantom limb'. Someone experiencing the latter knows exactly where the natural limb should be even though it is no longer there. To guard against 'phantom limb' it is important for sections of the artificial limb to be placed where the wearer feels they should be.

A small number of people who undergo amputation feel 'phantom pain'—that is, pain in the limb that is no longer there. The cause of the sensation is still being researched.

Q Does the wearing of an artificial limb cause any unpleasant odour?

A The socket of the artificial limb fits very closely to the stump of the natural one, and at the place where they meet the body may perspire. There will be no unpleasant smell of sweat if the wearer of the artificial limb is careful about personal hygiene, about keeping the limb itself thoroughly clean and about wearing a 'stump sock', which can be washed daily.

Q My son was born with one arm and needs an artificial limb. Will it be heavier than a natural limb and tire him out?

A The weight of an artificial limb is only about one-fifth of that of a natural limb, but because the latter is totally attached to the body, its weight is not obvious. A light but badly fitting artificial limb may feel heavier than one that is actually heavier but well fitting because the wearer will be conscious of it. So you need not be anxious about the weight of your son's artificial arm—if it is properly fitted it will not tire him.

Modern artificial limbs are highly efficient, comfortable and inoffensive to look at—and they are specially adapted to meet the individual needs of wearers.

An artificial limb is the product of highly skilled design and engineering, based on detailed and constantly improving research into the structure of the human frame and the movements of which it is capable, from walking and running to the slightest bending of a finger joint.

This limb must not simply fill the gap left by a missing natural limb or part of a limb, but must work comfortably and efficiently, so that it is as complete a replacement as possible, in both appearance and function.

Care in design

Amputation or the malformation of a natural limb at birth may cause the need for an artificial limb. Whatever the reason for it, it will be made according to precise and detailed information about the person who will use it: about age, height, weight and the general structure of the body, balance, skin colour and the way in which the person customarily makes movements and gestures.

The design of the limb will also take into consideration the way of life of the person concerned, particularly in terms of work and the things he or she enjoys doing in leisure time.

Comfort and efficiency

However well an artificial limb may be designed, its success as a useful addition to the body will obviously depend upon the attitude of the person who uses it. This in turn depends mainly upon two things: comfort and acceptance.

The design of modern, natural-looking artificial limbs takes into account all aspects of a person's life.

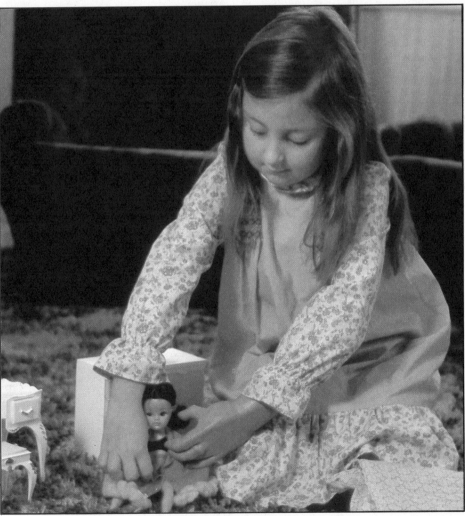

'Mother' Magazine

It is essential for an artificial limb to be comfortable. In its design and construction, great care is taken to ensure that the remaining part of the natural limb (the 'stump') and the 'socket' of the artificial one fit together smoothly. If there is no irritation or awkwardness in movement, the new limb will be accepted and become thoroughly useful much more quickly.

Good design and construction can do a great deal to make an artificial limb comfortable to wear and to use. How well it functions in use depends, first and foremost, upon a very detailed study of human movement, gesture and general physical behaviour.

Complexity of movement

It is easier to replace certain parts of the body with artificial limbs than others. The hand, for example, can make many small, delicate gestures; an artificial hand cannot, by itself, carry out more than a few of them, but is so constructed that a whole range of skilfully designed devices can be fitted to it so that the wearer can carry out precise and complex movements, such as those involved in driving a car.

The movements of the hip and knee are, by comparison with those of the hand, much more restricted, and an artificial limb can therefore replace them so accurately that the person wearing it will move in a natural way.

Training

No matter how well an artificial limb is designed, it can only function successfully if the person using it accepts it without fear or embarrassment and finds satisfaction in making it work to the full extent of its design. Both acceptance and adeptness depend, to some extent, on training. Anyone who needs to wear an

This detail of the car shows the modified control panel fitted into the right-hand door for ease of movement.

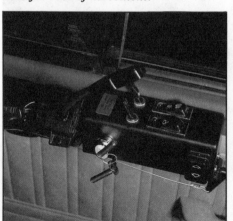

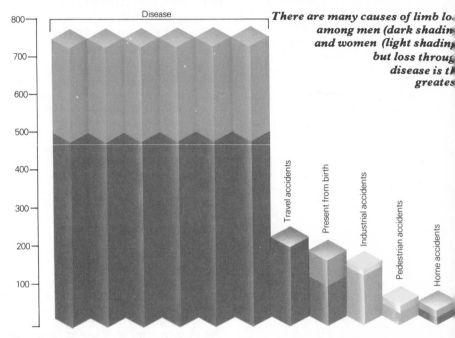

Causes of limb loss in the UK within one year

There are many causes of limb lo... among men (dark shadin... and women (light shading... but loss throug... disease is t... greates...

Disease

Travel accidents

Present from birth

Industrial accidents

Pedestrian accidents

Home accidents

artificial limb—and there are many thousands of people who do—can have expert help from specially trained staff in a number of major hospitals.

An artificial limb is an addition to the body, something imposed upon it, often after the shock of amputation, and the person who wears it must have time and

encouragement to grow accustomed to in his thoughts and emotions as well as use it to its best advantage and witho... self-consciousness.

This car has been specially adapted for thalidomide victim. Note the steering wheel extended to reach her arms.

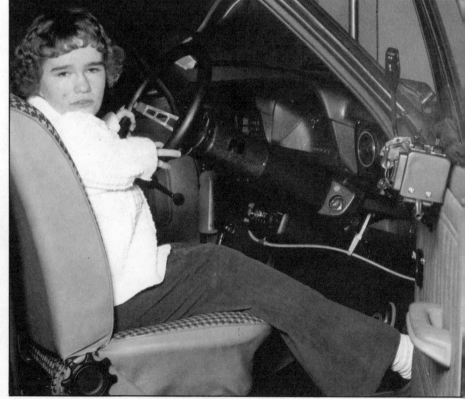

Nelson Hargreaves

Artificial respiration

Q Could I be asphyxiated if I fell asleep in front of my gas fire and the flame went out?

A Unfortunately this is possible, although the likelihood depends on the size of your room. As the air in the room becomes filled with gas, the amount of oxygen reaching your lungs will decrease. In the end you would become unconscious and die. To help prevent an accident like this, never sleep in front of the fire if it is on a low flame and make sure your room is draught-proof. Alternatively, use an electric convector heater, which is much safer.

Q My mother told me that it is very dangerous to give some kinds of foods to toddlers because it's possible they may choke on them. Is this true?

A Yes. Because they have not learned to chew properly, you do have to take care what you give to a child who is under three, especially if they are unsupervised for any length of time.

Never give hard sweets, pieces of apple, or any food in large chunks that could be difficult to swallow, and possibly cause an obstruction. Peanuts are the most dangerous of all, because there is a high risk that they will be swallowed whole. If this happens and a peanut gets lodged in the child's windpipe, turn him or her upside down and slap the back to dislodge it. If a peanut has reached the lungs, get the child to hospital as soon as possible. If the child's breathing stops, it is crucial to give mouth-to-mouth artificial respiration immediately.

Q When she has a temper tantrum, my little girl holds her breath until she goes blue in the face. Could she suffocate by doing this?

A No, because eventually the mechanisms of the body come into operation to start her breathing again—although this may not happen until she has lost consciousness for a few seconds. To stop the attack before it reaches this stage, try hooking your index finger over her tongue and pulling the tongue forward. This will make her take a breath.

Everyone should know how to give artificial respiration because it could save a life in an emergency.

Artificial respiration is the most important first aid technique for the relief of asphyxia. Asphyxia literally means 'absence of pulse', but is used to describe suffocation. A person who is suffocating is suffering from a lack of oxygen, which is normally obtained from breathing in the air. The victim struggles for breath and if this fight is unsuccessful, unconsciousness follows.

Causes of asphyxia

Oxygen is essential to keep the body alive and working and is carried to all parts via the bloodstream; a deficiency can have many causes. Air may not be able to get in and out of the nose and mouth because they are covered by a plastic bag, a pillow, or some other obstruction such as a sleeping cat in a baby's crib or pram. Or the airway between mouth and lungs may be blocked by food that has gone down the 'wrong way', a toy, the victim's tongue, broken or false teeth, or vomit. The airway can also be closed through swelling caused by swallowing scalding or corrosive liquid, or by an insect sting.

Any constriction of the neck, as in strangulation, has the same result. Sometimes the windpipe closes up naturally; this could happen because of noxious gases or through diseases such as bronchitis and asthma. Crushing of the chest, a common injury in car and crowd accidents, is another way in which the airway can be blocked.

Methods of artificial respiration

In the 'kiss of life', you take a deep breath, and after firmly sealing your lips over those of the victim, breathe out firmly.

Even if the airway is clear, the body may still become deprived of oxygen. The air breathed in may contain carbon monoxide which will be absorbed by the tissues in place of oxygen. Cyanide (prussic acid) fumes can render the body incapable of using oxygen. Air full of smoke, gas or dust is low in oxygen and, if breathed in, can result in asphyxia.

The air at high altitude is 'thin' in oxygen and has the same effect. Respiration will also stop, bringing on asphyxia, if the nerves that control breathing are injured by electrocution, pesticides, excessive use of drugs such as morphia or barbiturates, or by the spinal cord being crushed.

Effects of asphyxia

Whatever its cause, the outcome of this lack of oxygen is the same. Breathing becomes deeper and more rapid as the body tries to compensate for the oxygen deficiency. At the same time, the heartbeat – and the pulse – speed up as the body desperately tries to get more oxygen to the tissues.

As the blood's oxygen content goes down, its carbon dioxide content rises and it turns from bright red to a bluish-purple. This change is reflected in the skin which turns blue, particularly in the face, neck and at the extremities (the hands and feet).

As the blood is increasingly deprived of oxygen, the brain ceases to function fully and the victim loses consciousness. When this happens, the brain may 'misfire', causing seizures and foaming at the mouth. Finally, respiration will fail and soon afterwards the heart follows.

Life-saving action

Asphyxia is an emergency that demands drastic life-saving measures. Artificial respiration is most important as it not only gets breathing started again, but also increases the oxygen in the blood, which helps prevent permanent injury to the brain. The brain will suffer irreversible damage if it is totally starved of oxygen for a period lasting more than about four minutes.

Everyone should know how to give artificial respiration – when an accident occurs there is no time to look up the instructions in a book. But do not rush in and start artificial respiration without thinking first. If a room is filled with carbon monoxide or some other poisonous gas, it is essential to open the doors or windows first; if not, you too will soon be asphyxiated. In the case of electrocution it is vital to switch off the current before touching the victim. Should the asphyxia be caused by choking, try to dislodge any deep obstruction immediately.

Methods of artificial respiration

Mouth-to-mouth artificial respiration for an adult

You must be quick but careful. Learn this routine by heart in case you have to use it in an emergency when there is neither time nor opportunity to look up instructions in a book. Always make sure that clothing is loosened and the airway is clear before starting artificial respiration, but do not bother to try to drain the water from the lungs of someone who has drowned—this is a waste of precious time as there is no chance of removing the water completely. Points to remember during mouth to mouth resuscitation are to watch the victim's chest as you breathe into the lungs to make sure they are filling with air and to look for a fall in the chest as you take your mouth away. For maximum effect give the first five breaths as quickly as possible then aim for a rhythm of one breath every five seconds. Between breaths call for help if you are alone. If feasible try to pull the victim towards a window between breaths to get fresh air. Ask any onlookers to loosen any other tight clothing and to cover the victim with a coat or blanket. Most important of all, keep going.

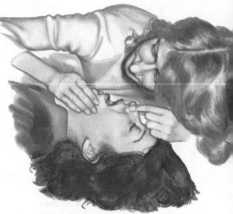

Put one hand under the chin and the other on the forehead so that your finger and thumb can reach the nose. Send any onlooker for help.

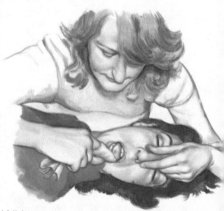

With one hand pinch the nose shut. Check the airway and remove any obstructions such as food, vomit or dentures by sweeping one finger round the mouth.

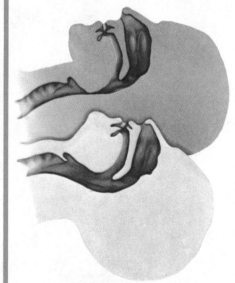

Turn the victim on his or her back and tilt the head back as far as possible so that the tongue falls against the palate and the airway is clear. Very quickly loosen any tight clothing at neck or waist.

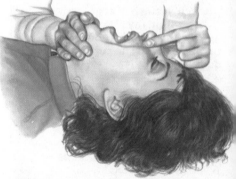

Administer the 'kiss of life' (see previous page). Now take your mouth away and watch the chest sink. Breathe in again and give five breaths quickly.

Mouth-to-mouth artificial respiration for a baby or child.

The rules for giving mouth-to-mouth artificial respiration to a child are exactly as for an adult but it is important not to breathe out too hard as this may over-inflate the lungs.

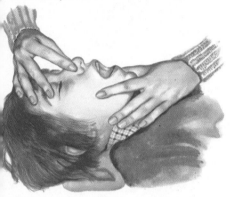

Clear the airway as for an adult, pinch the nose and take a shallow breath.

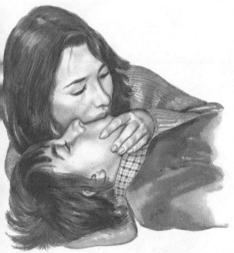

Breathe out very gently. For a very small child breathe into the nose and mouth.

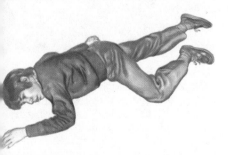

If the child starts to breathe, place him or her in the recovery position as shown.

The Silvester method

The Silvester method of artificial respiration should be used only as an alternative to the mouth-to-mouth method when an accident victim has facial injuries which make it impossible to place your mouth over the victim's, or because strong poison has been swallowed which could affect you as well, or if there is profuse vomiting, in which case the mouth-to-mouth method could cause choking by pushing vomit into the bronchial tubes and lungs. When using this method make sure that the support is under the victim's shoulders, not beneath the neck, so that the head can be bent back as far as possible for maximum clearance of the airway. As you press down on the victim's chest, make sure that you press on the lungs, not on the abdomen, which could damage internal organs. For a child press lightly to avoid internal damage.

Place the victim on his or her back on a firm surface. Put a cushion or folded blanket under the shoulders and push the head back. Kneel at the head with your knees either side of the forehead, then grasp the wrists and press them on the chest.

For an adult, press down with your whole body weight, then lean back on to your heels, still grasping the victim's wrists, so that the arms move in a wide arc and the hands are on the ground. Repeat once every five seconds.

Protecting your child from suffocation: some common hazards to avoid

Age	Risk	Preventive action
Birth to one year	**Choking**—on milk that is 'brought back'	Lie baby on front or side, not back. Never leave alone, feeding from propped-up bottle
	swallowing small object	Keep beads, buttons, marbles out of reach. Ensure soft toys have 'safety' eyes
	Suffocation—pillow falling on face	Do not give baby a pillow. Do not sleep with baby in your bed. If propping up child, put pillow under mattress
	plastic sticking to face	Cover plastic-lined baby carriage or crib sides with loosely-woven cotton fabric e.g. muslin. Remove plastic cover from mattress. Keep spare plastic pants out of reach
One year upwards	cat going to sleep on baby's face	Do not keep cat, alternatively fit cat net on crib and baby carriage
	Suffocation—plastic bag on head	Keep polyethylene bags out of reach. Knot ends of bag
	child climbing into old refrigerator	Remove door or use chain and padlock – better still, get refuse department to remove
	gas turned on	Fit fire-guard, have self-igniting type
	Drowning	Never leave toddler alone in bath; water must be shallow enough for child to be able to raise head when lying face down
		Cover ponds with wire mesh—better still fill in. Empty paddling pools after use
		Accompany child when paddling. Do not allow near rivers, lakes etc. without adults accompanying. Teach to swim as early as possible
	Electric shock	Be firm about not touching plugs
		Use safety plugs with shuttered sockets. Fit dummy plugs on unused sockets
		Do not give child electric blanket
		Check all appliances for wiring and earthing
		Avoid toys that are powered from wall sockets

For an adult, quickly roll the victim on to his or her side and give several short, sharp slaps between the shoulder blades. For a child, turn upside down and slap on the back. Do not bother to try tipping the water from someone who has drowned—start artificial respiration immediately. Always use the 'kiss of life' or mouth-to-mouth method unless the victim has severe facial injuries (in which case use the Silvester method, as illustrated).

Points to remember

Always give the first five breaths as quickly as possible, to get a surge of oxygen into the blood and help prevent irreversible brain damage.

Do not blow too hard or the lungs may be damaged and air may get into the stomach, possibly causing vomiting.

If efforts seem to be useless because the airway from the mouth is completely blocked, try blowing air in through the victim's nose.

Keep a close watch on the heart. If it stops beating, get someone to start heart massage at 60 pressures a minute, or intersperse 15 pressures on the heart with two quick mouth-to-mouth breaths.

Most important of all, keep going—someone's life may depend on it.

Even against seemingly insuperable odds, the victim will usually respond to artificial respiration and start to breathe. When this starts it may be shallow, or breaths may come in intermittent gasps.

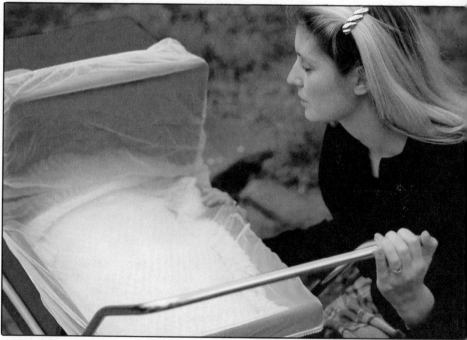

A net on the baby's carriage deters cats from entering it and lying on the child, causing suffocation.

Stop to allow the patient a chance to breathe on his or her own, but if breathing is spasmodic give an extra small breath or two to help restore the normal breathing pattern.

Once the patient is breathing properly, turn him or her on to one side into the recovery position with the leg and arm bent; the other side of the body should be straight with the head facing towards the bent arm. The chin should tilt down so that any vomit can easily drain from the mouth. Unless it has been impossible to call for help until now, do not leave the victim on any account until emergency help arrives on the scene.

Asbestosis

Q Since reading about asbestosis, I have realized that the iron-rest on my ironing board is made of asbestos. Am I in any danger?

A No, not really. An advisory committee on the use of asbestos in household goods has reported that the general public is in little danger. The material has to be in a fibrous state before it can be inhaled and cause damage. The asbestos used on ironing boards is compressed and so is quite safe; but once it starts to disintegrate, it should be thrown away.

Q Is there any risk in drinking water that has passed through cement-impregnated asbestos pipes?

A No. Surveys of areas where these type of pipes have been in use for many years, show that there is no excess risk of cancers of the bowel or abdomen.

Q Do those who work with asbestos bring the dust home and put their families at risk?

A This did happen occasionally in the past, when workers used to come home wearing their dusty overalls and workclothes straight from the factory floor. Nowadays, however, they are required to change their clothing and shower before coming home, so there is little chance of asbestos dust being brought into the home.

Q I am thinking of taking a job that involves handling asbestos. Will my employers spell out the risks, and how can I protect myself?

A Begin by asking your future employers to supply you with all the various government pamphlets on the subject; these should tell you what you need to know. If they are a responsible company, they should offer training courses to all employees, explaining the nature of asbestosis and suggesting ways in which you can protect yourself. They should also provide protective clothing and masks and offer facilities to their employees for washing or showering.

Research shows that asbestos can cause severe lung disease. As a result, those working with it are protected by strict regulations and regular medical checks.

Asbestosis is the name given to the lung disease caused by the mineral asbestos. It most commonly affects people who, in the course of their work, have to handle the substance and are unable to avoid breathing in its microscopic fibres from the air.

Asbestos is an unusual mineral because it is naturally fibrous. It has proved useful for years because the fibres, after being extracted from the ore after mining, can be woven or compressed into a material that is heat-and fire-resistant. This makes it invaluable in the manufacture of textiles, for brake and clutch linings, and in the building industry, for boarding, piping, insulation, use in paints and as tiles.

The disease

Since asbestos was first used commercially towards the end of the 19th century, its ill effects have been noted. It only affects those people who work with the mineral which, when inhaled can cause fibrosis of the lungs (thickening of lung tissues). Minor forms of the disease are only detectable through chest X-rays.

Symptoms of asbestosis include a noticeable shortening of breath, a lack of oxygen in the blood that leads to the familiar 'blueness' known as cyanosis and the thickening of the ends of the fingers, called 'clubbing'.

Unfortunately, asbestos fibres can also cause cancer; they are able to penetrate the cells of the body, which can ultimately lead to cancer developing. Those directly related to asbestos exposure which affect the lining membrane of the lung or abdomen are lung cancer and cancers of the stomach and bowel.

This lung cancer is the same type as is caused by smoking, and asbestos workers who smoke are especially vulnerable.

The tumours are particularly related to exposure to blue asbestos, of which there is still a lot in lagging and buildings. So care has to be taken when replacing it or in demolition work.

Evidence concerning cancer of the bowel is less conclusive, but it would appear that workers who face contamination are certainly at risk.

Prevention

Ignorance about the effects of asbestos has caused great suffering in the past. In fact, tumours are still occurring that can be traced back to contamination 30 to 40 years ago.

Nowadays, the dangers are recognized and workers are protected by law. Strict regulations are laid down about working conditions, the provision of protective clothing and the wearing of masks, the monitoring of levels of asbestos in the air, and facilities for washing and showering.

Workers who deal with asbestos wear protective clothing and masks.

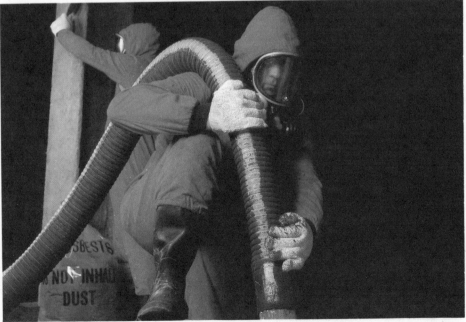

Courtesy of Envirocor Ltd

Aspirin and analgesics

Q Do painkillers act as sleeping tablets?

A Strictly speaking, no. Milder painkillers may help by relieving pain which has been disrupting sleep. Some of the stronger ones obtainable on prescription do also act as sedatives and can induce sleep.

Q I am taking an analgesic. Is it safe for me to drink alcohol?

A If you're using a mild analgesic—aspirin or acetaminophen, say—there should be no problem in taking an occasional drink. However, both aspirin and undiluted spirits can cause bleeding in the gut, so it is wise to avoid the combination if you have a delicate stomach.

Alcohol is a good standby for severe pain, but it should never be taken at the same time as a strong painkiller because both substances slow down breathing and the interaction of the two substances could be dangerous.

Q My husband gets bad migraines; if he doesn't get treatment straight away it always takes a long time for them to go. Why is this?

A What happens is that when a migraine attack occurs, the body shuts down the stomach. Once this happens, there is little chance of any drug being absorbed—so make sure your husband gets treatment immediately or his chances of a rapid recovery will be reduced. If this is impossible for any reason, your doctor may prescribe an analgesic in suppository form, or administer a drug orally that will assist absorption.

Q Can aspirin work as a male contraceptive pill?

A This is not as unlikely as it sounds, but the doses must be very large. Aspirin inhibits the production of prostaglandins, which are associated with sperm production. In an American study of analgesic abuse, few men became fathers while taking large doses of aspirin. But in animal tests, large doses caused their testicles to shrink and inhibited sperm production. Obviously, aspirin is an unreliable contraceptive.

There are many analgesics—or painkillers—easily available today, of which aspirin is the most widely advertised, but it is important to know the right analgesic to take to relieve a particular pain.

The range of pain-killing drugs available can be confusing. Some are fairly mild, some are dangerous; many can be bought at drugstores or supermarkets, others obtained only on prescription.

The commonest analgesic is aspirin. It is used for ailments ranging from flu to fevers, from period pains to rheumatism, and is also, of course, the much heralded standby for 'tension headache'.

However, aspirin is not suitable for pain connected with the heart, gut or urinary tract, or for those who may develop rashes and breathing difficulties with it. Neither would acetaminophen, another popular analgesic, be good for some people with liver trouble. If in any doubt, ask in the drugstore for a suitable product. If pain persists, don't just take more pills; see your doctor.

Painkillers in action

Pain is transmitted (A) by prostaglandins across synapses (gaps between a nerve ending and a new nerve beginning), along the nerves, and finally to the brain. Painkillers act (B) by inhibiting the production of prostaglandins.

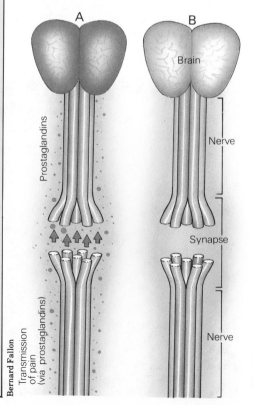

Bernard Fallon
Transmission of pain (via prostaglandins)

Prostaglandins

A

B

Brain

Nerve

Synapse

Nerve

Dosage
As a general rule, take a painkiller befor pain really gets bad; use enough for it work, but don't go over the suggeste dose. With aspirin, this is 4gm, or 12 ta lets, in 24 hours, or double that for acu rheumatism. Recent research has show that it is unsafe to administer aspirin children under twelve years old.

Types
Analgesics fall into one of two cat gories—those that act locally on a specif pain, and those that act centrally, fro within, and which affect the who nervous system.

The first group of analgesics which ar known as peripheral painkillers, includ aspirin, acetaminophen and the onc popular phenacetin—now no longer use because of its effect on the kidneys. A these are used to relieve mild to moderat pain in muscles, joints or bones, and the work by reducing the body's production substances called prostaglandins whic cause muscles to contract, so making th person more susceptible to pain.

The centrally-acting painkillers ar much more powerful and are therefor more strictly controlled by law. Th category includes codeine, DF118 an distalgesic. It also covers all the opiate whether natural or synthetic, an includes morphine and heroin as well a opium itself.

Opiates work by dulling pain throug interacting with the brain's ow naturally produced morphine-lik substances called endorphins. They ar all inclined to produce side-effects suc as slowing breathing, nausea, vomitin, constipation and – most serious of all tolerance and addiction.

Codeine is also an opiate, and becaus of this, you can only obtain it with prescription.

Alternatives
It is also worth noting that analgesic are not the only way to relieve pai Non-chemical methods such as applyin cold water (for burns and bruises to th skin) or heat and massage (for painfu aching muscles) can bring relief, whil techniques on the fringes of orthodo medicine such as acupuncture, electrica stimulation, meditation and biofeedbac are well worth trying in mild as well a really chronic cases.

Painkillers—their uses and effects

Drug	Used for	Effects
Aspirin	Acute or chronic aches and pains (e.g. tension headache, period pains, neuralgia, toothache); flu; fevers; rheumatism	Fast-acting; reduces fever and inflammation; does not cause dependence in users. Can irritate stomach, affect hearing and cause rashes and breathing problems in some people
Acetaminophen	Aches and pains; flu; fevers	Reduces fever; no gastric irritation. Does not reduce inflammation. Effects less prolonged than aspirin. Constant use can affect liver function
Codeine	Aches and pains; coughs; mild diarrhoea	Slightly constipating; in large doses can slow down breathing and cause nausea
Phenylbutazone	Rheumatic and joint disorders	Reduces inflammation and swelling. Can cause fluid retention, nausea and blood disorders
Morphine	Diarrhoea (with kaolin as liquid mixture); severe pain (e.g. in injuries, heart attack, coronary thrombosis, after surgery)	Swift and effective. Can cause constipation, nausea, slow breathing. Derived from opium and therefore addictive

DOs and DON'Ts of pain relief

DO
- take a painkiller soon after the pain begins, otherwise it will be more difficult to relieve it.
- find out how painkillers interact with any other medicines being taken.
- take painkillers with food or milk to reduce the risk of stomach irritation.
- give children smaller doses, as indicated on the label. If in doubt, ask the chemist about the correct dosage. Soluble painkillers are best for children; mix them in fruit juice or milk.
- buy medicines in childproof bottles and keep all drugs out of their reach
- induce vomiting if you suspect an overdose. Drinking salty water or thrusting two fingers down the throat usually brings it on.

DON'T
- take painkillers often or in large doses without medical advice.
- take more than the stated dose
- store painkillers, especially aspirin, in the bathroom or anywhere moist—they will perish. A cool, dry place is best.

Di Lewis

Asthma

Q Is there anything I can do if I forget my inhaler and then suffer an attack?

A There is very little you can do and this sort of situation only serves to emphasize how important it is to carry your medication with you always. If you suffer a severe attack then you must go to a doctor or a hospital emergency department as soon as possible. In the meantime it is most important that you sit still and save your breath.

Q My father had asthma when he was a lad and my son and I have it. Can asthma run in families?

A Unfortunately, asthma does have a tendency to run in families, especially those asthmas which are a strong response to an allergy. The inherited link is not yet fully understood.

Q I use an inhaler for my asthma about five or six times a day. But I've heard that the inhaler is dangerous for the heart. Is this true?

A No. Bronchodilator inhalers had a bad reputation some years ago because they over-stimulated the heart. Modern inhalers affect the heart much less and so are far safer.

Q My two young children are both asthmatic, but they are also full of energy. Should they be allowed to play sports?

A Definitely yes. Any asthmatic should be vigorously encouraged to participate in sport. Some sports may be more likely to cause asthma than others, and in this case the child should make sure that he has his inhaler handy. Of all sports, swimming is the least likely to bring on an attack.

Q Why does my son always seem to get an asthmatic attack when we have guests?

A There is often a connection between emotional stress and asthma attacks. Try to make your son feel more relaxed. Involve him in the preparations, and avoid pushing him into the limelight.

Asthma is a very common respiratory complaint—so it is essential to know the symptoms, the treatments available and the ways of preventing an attack.

Asthma involves a severe narrowing of the bronchial tubes. These lead from the windpipe—called the trachea—into the lungs and they carry the oxygen we breathe in to all parts of the lungs and provide a path for the carbon dioxide (a waste product of the body) to escape up the trachea when we breathe out.

The narrowing of the bronchial tubes—or bronchi—results from the contraction of the muscle lining them and causes difficulty in breathing that is most marked when breathing out. For this reason, asthmatics tend to breathe in in short gasps and breathe out with a long wheeze—a result of the effort required to breathe against the obstruction.

The body's defences

Two different chemicals are responsible for causing the bronchial muscles to contract. One is histamine, which is released from mast cells (cells that store histamine) as part of an allergic reaction and the other is acetyl choline which is a chemical released from the nerve endings which control the bronchial muscle.

These nerves are branches of the important vagus nerve which originates in the brain. The vagus keeps the bronchi in a constant state of contraction all the time and, as such, can be regarded as the main control over bronchial contraction with additional control being provided by histamine.

To keep the balance between contraction and expansion (dilation), there are other substances that cause the bronchi to relax, thus working against the histamine and acetylcholine. These substances are called bronchodilators and a number of them are manufactured in the adrenal glands situated above each kidney.

The most important bronchodilator is adrenalin, which acts as a stimulant during periods of stress and excitement when we need more oxygen to provide energy during a dangerous situation, the adrenalin helps to open up the bronchi to allow more air through to the lungs during rapid breathing.

In addition to this, the bronchial muscles also contain enzymes—substances which are responsible for maintaining certain bodily functions on which life depends; among these is respiration (breathing)—and these help to protect them from the action of histamine and acetyl choline.

The use of an inhaler containing a drug such as ventolin gives almost immediate relief from an asthmatic attack.

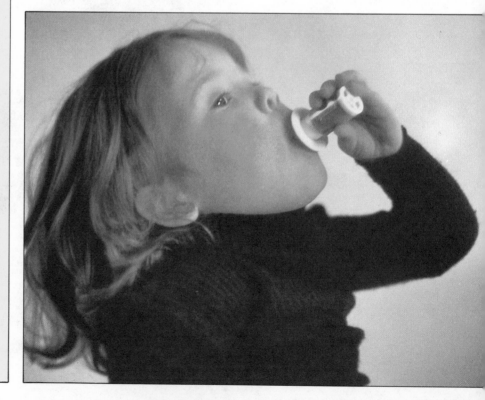

The respiratory system

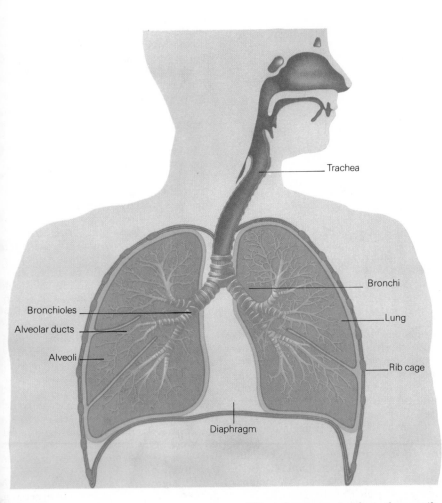

The respiratory system diagram labels:
- Trachea
- Bronchi
- Lung
- Rib cage
- Bronchioles
- Alveolar ducts
- Alveoli
- Diaphragm

We also know that emotional upsets or anxiety may occasionally worsen an asthmatic condition, though how this happens is not clear.

Unknown causes

Unfortunately, there are a number of causes of asthma which are not fully understood. For certain people, asthma frequently occurs after vigorous exercise, especially running. It is probable that both histamine and the vagus nerve are involved, though, generally speaking, the more vigorous the running and the cooler the air which is breathed, the worse the asthma becomes.

Certain drinks, foods and preservatives can also produce an asthmatic response. Rather than being a straightforward allergic response, it is often the result of the body's sensitivity to certain substances. Again, the mechanism involved is still not fully understood.

Symptoms

The typical asthma attack is characterized by a sudden shortness of breath and wheezing, which is sometimes accompanied by coughing. The bringing up of phlegm is not a prominent part of the attack and suggests that the patient may also have bronchitis. Generally speaking, asthmatics are more prone to chest infections, and this is caused by a failure to clear the lungs fully. Many patients often develop a hunched look which is brought about by the constant effort of breathing.

In many cases, the onset of asthma follows a seasonal pattern as the pollen count rises. This pattern is often accompanied by irritations to the nose and sneezing, which we usually refer to as hay fever.

Of course, allergies to house pets and the house mite will occur all through the year as the allergen is constantly in the

The microscopic house mite, present in dust and bedding, can trigger an attack.

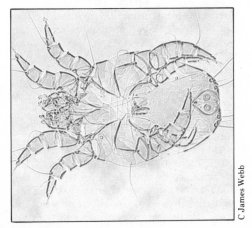

Causes

Asthma is brought on by a number of different causes, ranging from breathing polluted air to emotional upset, which makes it a rather complex problem to treat. However, since all the causes of asthma trigger the release of either histamine or acetyl choline, it is important to understand these two chemical reactions in order to see why people are vulnerable to asthma.

Histamine release is the most common cause of asthma, and the process which brings it about is rather remarkable considering that the substances which trigger it—house dust containing house mites, animal fur, pollen and fungal spores among others—are so varied.

Some people develop an excessive amount of an antibody (a protein made by the body as part of its defence system) to some substances breathed in—these substances (some of which are listed above) are known as allergens and they cause allergic reactions. It is this malfunction of the body's defences which starts the reaction leading to asthma.

What happens is that the antibody, which is known as immunoglobulin E, or IgE, attaches itself to the mast cells where the histamine is stored. The next time the allergen is inhaled, each molecule (particles which make up the whole antibody) of IgE pairs up with a neighbouring molecule and, as a result of this mating, the mast cell releases its store of histamine. The bronchi then begins to contract, making it increasingly difficult to breathe: the condition that we call asthma.

Acetyl choline released from the nerve endings in the bronchial tubes can be caused by a number of substances which irritate both the bronchial tubes and the nerve endings. These nerve endings then send messages to the vagus with the information that they have been irritated. In response, the vagus nerve then contracts the bronchial muscles and so starts asthmatic breathing difficulties. The same sort of irritation is caused by viral or bacterial infections of the throat, which explains why asthma tends to get worse with chest infections and colds.

C James Webb

Asthma: its causes and prevention

Although an asthmatic condition must always be treated with drugs and according to the doctor's advice, there are some preventive measures that can be taken.

Causes	Preventive measures
INFECTIONS: common cold, some viral infections, sinusitis, bronchitis	Avoid groups and individuals with colds; stick to balanced diet, have adequate sleep, take moderate exercise
ALLERGENS BREATHED IN: pollens, house dust, feathers, fungal spores, animal hair	Keep house as dust-free as possible. Use foam pillows; avoid animals; fit electronic air cleaners
IRRITANTS BREATHED IN: fumes, like tobacco smoke, paint fumes; air pollutants; cold air	Avoid all fumes; stop smoking and avoid smokers; avoid going out into cold air
FOOD ALLERGENS: Can include milk, eggs, strawberries, fish, tomatoes	Isolate allergen through prick test and then avoid it
PSYCHOLOGICAL CHANGES: stress, emotional disturbance	Reduce or eliminate causes of stress; stop worrying, and avoid emotional disturbance
TRIGGER MECHANISMS: physical exertion; sudden changes in temperature	Avoid sudden physical exertion; approach exercise in relaxed manner; avoid constant temperature changes
DRUGS: Can include penicillin, vaccines, anaesthetics	Identify drugs that cause allergic reaction and avoid them. There are alternatives available

air. The house mite is particularly keen on living in warm places, like beds, and for this reason asthma attacks often seem to happen at night. In fact, coughing at night in children may well be a result of this allergy.

Treatment
The treatment given for asthma largely depends on the type of asthma and the severity of the attacks, but it is broadly divided into two: emergency treatment for severe attacks, requiring a visit from the doctor or admission to hospital, and everyday self-medication to prevent an attack occurring, which is known as prophylactic, or preventive, treatment and can be carried out at home.

The aim of emergency treatment is to bring relief as rapidly as possible and so one of three drugs is given by injection: adrenalin, aminophylline and hydro-cortisone, and these have an almost instantaneous effect. The first two act directly on the bronchial muscles, raising the enzyme level and so relaxing the muscle. The third is a steroid, and although it acts quickly to relieve the attack, how it works is not known. In very severe cases, oxygen may also be given to the patient.

Most asthmatics take some form of daily treatment, usually in the form of tablets or inhalers. The doctor will decide which type of drug is the most suitable after first diagnosing the cause of the asthma. To do this the prick test is used. This determines whether the asthma is a result of an allergic reaction and what the body is allergic to. A number of possible

allergens are introduced into the body through the skin. If the body reacts to any of these and produces a red weal, then the person is allergic to that particular allergen. A doctor may also measure the patient's breathing rate and capacity using a flow meter. This indicates just how much he or she is affected by the allergen.

Once the doctor has identified the most likely cause of the asthma he will prescribe the appropriate treatment. Wherever possible the allergen should be avoided. Drugs like intal—taken by inhalation—may be prescribed to decrease the release of histamine. Or a broncho-dilator, such as ventolin, taken either as

tablets or inhaled will give rapid rel from the effects of a sudden asthm attack, though not all people will react the drug with the same speed.

For those who suffer from a more pe sistent and severe form of asthm doctors may prescribe steroid drug Because of the side-effects of this type drug, patients will be asked to sti rigidly to the doctor's recommend dosage, and to make sure that th always have the drug with them in case an attack. The treatment should alwa be continued, as failure to do this ma encourage a further attack.

Prevention and outlook
Most asthmatics will have their conditi worsened or even triggered by everyda substances, and once the cause identified, the only course is to avoid it for instance, keeping the house as clear dust as possible, avoiding petrol fum and tobacco smoke, and also sudde exertion and emotional stress. There ar of course, many other irritants, but the are the more common ones that ca worsen an asthmatic condition.

However, it is difficult to be specific what affects one asthmatic may actual have a beneficial effect on another. But is accepted that regular, controlle exercise rather than sudden exertion do have a beneficial effect, and a asthmatics should be encouraged to tak as much regular—but strictly contro led—exercise as they can manage at an one time.

Although there is no absolute cure—5 per cent of child sufferers tend to grow ou of the complaint during adolescence asthmatics should be encouraged by th news that current research is producin positive results.

How histamine causes asthma

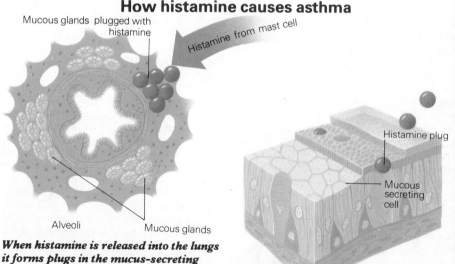

Mucous glands plugged with histamine

Histamine from mast cell

Alveoli

Mucous glands

Histamine plug

Mucous secreting cell

When histamine is released into the lungs it forms plugs in the mucus-secreting glands, which aggravates the glands and causes them to over-produce mucus.

Section through alveolar tissue

Astigmatism

Q I have noticed that my son often squints and narrows his eyes almost to a slit when he is watching television. Do you think it is possible that he might have an astigmatism?

A This is quite possible. Screwing the eyes up like this—which is simply a way of compensating for the distortion caused by astigmatism—is in fact one of the commonest signs used in the diagnosis of the condition.

You should take your son to the optometrist to have his eyes tested regularly. Astigmatism can be corrected satisfactorily with glasses. Do not delay, because poor sight may affect the child's progress at school.

Q For years now I have been wearing fairly strong glasses because I have an astigmatism and am also very short-sighted. But I like the idea of wearing contact lenses. Will this be possible with my eye condition?

A You would probably be able to wear hard contact lenses. These work by taking over the function of the cornea. Even severe astigmatism and 'irregular' corneal astigmatism can be corrected with the wearing of hard lenses.

The only kind of soft contact lenses which would be suitable for your astigmatism are those of a 'toric' design, which do not rotate on the eye and may be slightly thicker at the bottom. But even this kind of lens is not always satisfactory.

Q I suffer from astigmatism and am wondering if my children are at all likely to inherit the same problem.

A It is possible. For instance, if the rare condition of albinism—an absence of pigment that causes skin and hair to be white and the eyes to be unable to bear normal light or focus properly—exists in your family, you should consult your doctor as to the probability of your children inheriting the condition.

However, if your own astigmatism was caused by surgery or an injury, then your children will most certainly not inherit it.

Astigmatism is an eye condition which can cause blurred vision, headaches and fatigue. However, the right glasses or contact lenses can usually correct the problem.

If the curve of the front surface of the cornea, the outer covering of the eye, is irregular, the person will see a distorted image. This particular kind of sight defect is called astigmatism.

In fact, nearly everyone's eyes are affected to some extent by astigmatism, because very rarely does the front surface of the cornea provide a perfect lens. If the irregularity is slight, vision will not be noticeably affected. If it is marked, however, the image will be distorted—with vertical, horizontal or diagonal blurring, depending on the nature of the imperfection—and the condition will require treatment.

Causes
Astigmatism may be present from birth or it may develop in childhood over a number of years. Severe astigmatism may be inherited. Sometimes it is secondary to other eye conditions or it can result from the formation of scar tissue after the cornea has been diseased or injured. Or it may follow eye operations such as the removal of cataracts.

Occasionally, distortion may be caused by a part of the eye other than the cornea. Even slight dislocation of the lens inside the eye—for example, from a severe blow—will produce a warped image. So

will disease or pressure behind the eye affecting the fovea, the pinhead-sized area of the retina used for acute vision. But it is the cornea which is responsible for most cases.

Diagnosis and treatment
Astigmatism should be suspected in someone who narrows his or her eyelids almost to a slit in order to see more clearly. Diagnosis requires careful assessment of the irregularities of the cornea, testing with special patterns to determine exactly which part of the image is distorted and how severely. Instruments used to measure astigmatism include the retinoscope, which allows the light reflections from the inside of the eye to be studied, and the keratometer, which measures the corneal images.

Astigmatism is harder to correct than straightforward long or short sight. The commonest way is to prescribe glasses with cylindrical lenses ground to the required curvature, though the wearer may still notice some blurring. If, as often happens, astigmatism is accompanied by short or long sight, compound spectacle lenses are the answer.

Contact lenses may also be used, and very severe cases of 'irregular' astigmatism may call for a corneal graft.

Comparison of normal and astigmatic sight

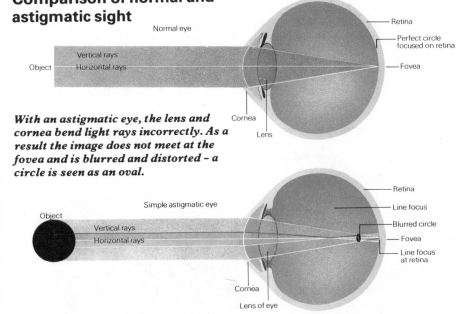

Normal eye

Object · Vertical rays · Horizontal rays · Cornea · Lens · Retina · Perfect circle focused on retina · Fovea

With an astigmatic eye, the lens and cornea bend light rays incorrectly. As a result the image does not meet at the fovea and is blurred and distorted – a circle is seen as an oval.

Simple astigmatic eye

Object · Vertical rays · Horizontal rays · Cornea · Lens of eye · Retina · Line focus · Blurred circle · Fovea · Line focus at retina

Hayward Art Group

Athlete's foot

Q I have a severe form of athlete's foot that keeps recurring. Is there any chance that the condition will leave my feet scarred or deformed?

A Thankfully, the fungus causing athlete's foot lives only on the superficial layers of the skin, eating dead skin cells. For this reason, there will be no scarring, but in chronic cases the nails may become affected and need specialist treatment with drugs. With correct treatment of skin and nails, the foot should return to normal.

Q I have grown weary of trying to get rid of athlete's foot. But every time I think it has gone for good, it makes a comeback. Is there a reason for this?

A The commonest reason for re-infection is that the fungus has never been properly eradicated in the first place. For this reason it is important to dust your shoes and socks, as well as your feet with antifungal powder as they can carry the fungus. It is also important to keep up the medical treatment for a considerable time after the symptoms have disappeared.

Q I have suffered from athlete's foot for some time now, and have just discovered a similar sort of irritation on my hands. Is it possible for athlete's foot to spread to other parts of the body?

A The athlete's foot fungus belongs to a group of fungi known as Trichophytons and these can live on various parts of the body. But they are not very contagious and so are unlikely to spread. However, there is a condition similar to athlete's foot that can affect the hands, and this should be diagnosed and treated by the doctor.

Q My daughter has athlete's foot. Can this spread to the rest of the family?

A Not if precautions are taken, the most important being hygiene; everyone should carefully wash and dry his or her own feet—with a personal towel—and use an antifungal powder on feet and shoes.

Athlete's foot is annoying and unpleasant, but usually responds well to treatment—and can be prevented.

Athlete's foot is a fungal infection and probably the most common foot complaint that doctors treat. It can affect almost everyone, though small children do appear to be immune.

Causes
The only real cause of athlete's foot is a failure to observe the necessary personal hygiene, along with carelessness in drying the feet after a bath. Those people who suffer from sweaty feet are particularly prone to this complaint and the situation can be aggravated by wearing airless, plastic shoes which prevent the feet from breathing.

It is the moist, sweaty areas between the toes that provide the soggy skin on which the fungus likes to settle. The fungus then lives on the skin, digesting the dead skin that the body sheds each day. Once the fungus starts eating the dead skin, it may then cause inflammation and damage to the living skin.

There is a small risk of picking up athlete's foot in bathrooms and in public changing rooms.

Symptoms and treatment
The first sign of athlete's foot is irritation and itching between the toes followed by the skin beginning to peel. This can be accompanied by bad foot odour.

In worse cases, painful red cracks, known as fissures, appear between the toes, and in the odd severe case, the toe-nails become affected. These become either soft or more brittle as the fungus invades the nail substance. It may be possible to see the nail thickening beneath its outer shell. In extreme cases, the foot swells and blisters—requiring prompt attention from the doctor.

Modern antifungal creams and powders are successful in the treatment of athlete's foot. Substances such as clotrimazole and tolnafate are extremely effective as creams or ointments, and need to be applied daily while the condition lasts, and for two or three weeks after the symptoms have disappeared to prevent its recurrence.

Where the infection is severe and the nails have been affected a drug known as griseofulvin may be prescribed by the doctor to be taken orally. It is effective within a few weeks. It is then necessary to dust the feet, socks and shoes with antifungal powder to prevent re-infection.

Athlete's foot can be treated at home, but if the problem begins to spread or refuses to respond to treatment then your doctor must be consulted.

Preventing athlete's foot
Chances of developing athlete's foot can be reduced by following a few guidelines on foot care.
* Wash the feet daily with soap, and clean all dirt from under the nails and between toes
* Dry each toe thoroughly with your own towel, paying particular attention to the gaps between toes
* Powder your feet with antifungal powder. To prevent re-infection also powder shoes
* Put on clean cotton or wool socks daily. Avoid nylon socks and plastic shoes. Wear open shoes if feet feel sweaty

---

The white, peeling skin of athlete's foot (left) can be treated with an antifungal powder (below). This can also be used to prevent infection where risk exists.

C James Webb

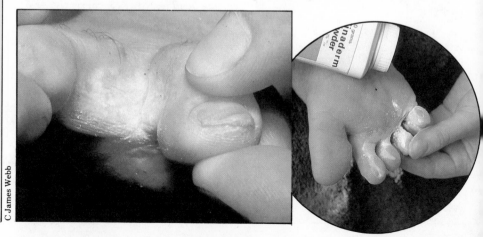

Attachment in infancy

Q My two-year-old son always clings to me whenever I take him to a children's party, though he is quite independent at home. Should I push him socially?

A Don't push him at all. In time, his confidence will increase and he will learn to cope with his shyness. Some children take quite a while to lose their reserve, and if you stay in the background at a party, you may eventually find there is a sudden burst of confidence.

Why not say at the beginning: 'Do you remember how much you enjoyed yourself last time? Well, I'll stay again this time, but if I see you are having a good time, I may slip out to do a bit of shopping; then I'll come back at the end.' This way, you should be able to leave without causing a disturbance and your child will be prepared.

Q I am going into hospital soon to have my second baby. Is there any way I can prepare my toddler for my absence?

A She is sure to miss you. And on your return you may find she either ignores you or becomes very demanding. All you can do is make sure things run smoothly while you are away and that she is looked after by someone she knows. Make sure it is someone you know and that she trusts. The more she becomes used to being handled by other people, the easier she will be able to cope with your absence.

Q In all the articles I read about attachment forming the emphasis is placed on the mother. Doesn't the father have a place? As an expectant 'dad', surely I can have as close a relationship with my baby as my wife?

A If this is what you want, then of course you can. Doctors seem to think that the baby forms the strongest attachment with the individual who looks after it most. So if you are going to share in the birth as much as you are able, and expect to share the responsibilities of your baby's everyday care, then it is likely that the bonding will be equally shared and you will be able to develop a close and loving relationship with your child.

It is important for a baby's emotional development that a loving attachment is formed with the mother – or whoever is to care for it – from birth. What, then, are the best ways of ensuring that this happens?

Babies have the ability to share a responsive and loving relationship from the moment they are born. But because of the way sexual roles are defined, a father may not be present at the birth, and the baby is first handed to the mother, making her the child's early contact.

Opinion is divided as to whether the strong bond that occurs between the mother and the infant is 'natural' or the result of conditioning from birth onwards. On the one hand, babies are said to respond more to the female voice, and that since it is women who are biologically equipped to bear children and breast-feed them, the bonding must be physiological. Others argue that attachment still occurs when a mother substitute takes over.

Bonding at birth

It is a common practice when a woman has given birth for the baby to be taken away, washed and wrapped in a blanket before being handed to the mother. Nowadays, some midwives are questioning this rather efficient, hygienic approach, and some hospitals are handing the newborn infant to the mother—often with the umbilical cord still attached – straight after the birth.

Medical evidence seems to suggest that this has important implications for the future and encourages the relationship between mother and baby.

Babies that experience early caressing, eye-to-eye contact, and the sound of their mother's voice in those few hours after the birth, appear to cry less, be more alert and responsive. Even later in their development, they appear to have a more relaxed relationship with their mothers and are more receptive, and their mothers more understanding.

Problems with bonding

Unfortunately, love is not something that you can turn on at will, and with some women the bonding can take longer to establish, or even prove absent altogether. The reasons for this are complex and varied, but can usually be traced back to the woman's own childhood and upbring-

Those moments after the birth are important for the baby and parents.

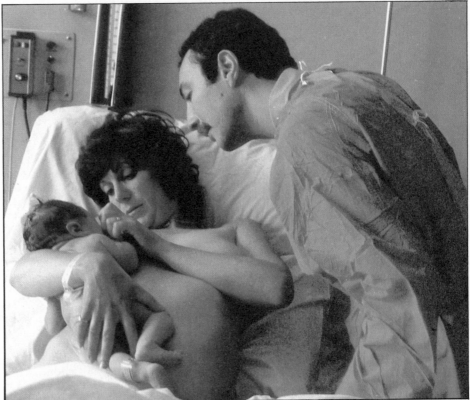

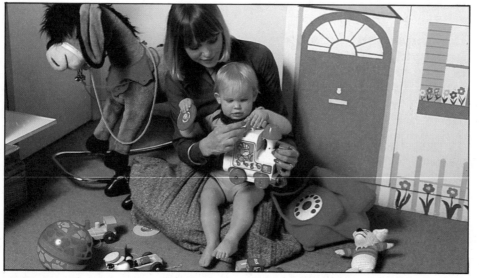

Di Lewis

A mother's close attention to her baby is essential to forming the early attachment so important for future development.

ing. She may have been unloved and neglected; she may fear handling such a small creature because of her own insecurity; or the baby simply may not be as appealing and attractive as she had hoped. A woman can suffer great conflict and unhappiness if her ideal of motherhood does not match up with the reality.

Health visitors are trained to recognize the negative feelings that mothers may display and provide encouragement and support. They may be able to put an unhappy mother in touch with a local self-help group that offers support to women in a state of post-natal depression.

Making the adjustment

A woman who is at ease with herself is more likely to be at ease with her baby. It is this loving acceptance that enables children to grow up and mature into secure adults.

Learning how to cope with your own emotions is also a basis for good mothering. For example, if you feel rising panic at the sound of your baby crying, stop what you are doing, take a few deep breaths and you will find that you become more relaxed and listen with a less acute feeling of anxiety. Sometimes you may have negative feelings of your own: anger, coldness, a lack of interest. It can be very wearisome to feel that you always have to respond to your child's every demand. You will soon learn to identify your baby's cries so that you can distinguish between a cry of hunger, a shriek of pain, a yell of impatience, a whimper of loneliness and the restless cry of the simply bored.

Giving attention

When you give your attention to your baby, give it wholly. Talk continually; the words may be meaningless but children will respond to the tone.

Not all the effort should be made by the mother, however. Babies respond just as happily to other adults, especially if they are used to them from the beginning. They are not only useful because they can lift some of the responsibility from the mother, but also because in forming a relationship with the baby they offer the beginnings of independence. Brothers and sisters can help in this way too.

Coping with clinging

All children cling to their mothers at some stage in their development. This usually happens between the ages of 18 months and three years. It takes the form of constant interruptions, creating a disturbance in a public place, and literally hanging on to mother's skirts.

This is an extremely trying stage, but there are two alternatives for solving the problems. First, you can give the attention as, when and where it is demanded, or you can give yourself a regular break by getting someone else to take over. Otherwise, find out where the nearest crèche is, to give your child the opportunity of being with other children of a similar age—and also give you a break.

Start the routine when the baby is under six months old, when it is more likely to adapt to new people.

Going back to work

Many mothers want to return to work when their babies are still small. Ideally, a good substitute mother should be provided, someone who will stay in your home and whose ideas on childrearing are similar to your own. Babies can adapt to substitute mothers without suffering

any obvious harm, and there is certain no proof that children of working mothe grow up any less well adjusted than tho of mothers who stay at home.

The moment of leaving a child inevitably traumatic. The baby ma initially cling or scream, causing th mother anguish and anxiety for the re of the day. The best thing to do is to sa goodbye firmly, with a confident smi and then to go without looking back ar ignore any wails of outrage.

Usually children adjust quickly. But the baby continues to cry, and afte several days is still not adjusting an even showing signs of fear or of becomin withdrawn, you may have to rethink you plan. Perhaps you have chosen the wron person or the wrong form of childcare; perhaps a single incident has triggere off such a response. In this case, it is tim for reassurance and a fresh start.

By the age of three, most childre recognize the fact that other children an the outside world are more interestin and can provide as much fun as mothe and father. They will go happily playschool, though it may be wise to sta this on a part-time basis. As they pla with other children and learn from othe adults, the ties will loosen. The bondin in terms of love and affection will remai with fewer strings attached.

Favourable factors

In hospital
● Holding the baby immediately after it is born
● Baby kept with mother; access at all times
● Breast-feeding (on demand, if required)
● Flexible visiting hours so father can be present as often as possible
● Good, sympathetic nursing; friendly, relaxed atmosphere
● Continual reassurance for mother and baby gained through cuddling, rocking, caressing

At home
● Good relationship between parents; loving, supportive father
● Continuing affection and reassurance
● Recognition of baby's individuality and need to develop resourcefulness
● Encouraging affection between baby and others, apart from parents
● Contact with other babies and children
● Ability of mother to 'let go', allowing baby to get to know other people and so develop independence

Autism

Autism is a distressing mental disability, but specialist teaching and a constructive approach can do much to help autistic children and adults.

Q I run a playschool and am wondering if one particularly noisy and undisciplined child might be autistic. At what age can you tell?

A Most easily between 2½ and 5 years, when the autistic pattern of behaviour becomes obvious. Since autism principally affects speech and social behaviour, it is almost impossible to detect during the first year of life. Some mothers of autistic babies sense that there is something wrong from birth, but cannot explain quite what it is that perturbs them.

Q My daughter is autistic, but my son seems perfectly normal. I am worried that he may become autistic—is this possible?

A Although the majority of autistic children have the condition from birth, some apparently normal young children have been known to become autistic after a severe illness or a highly upsetting experience. However, this fortunately does not happen very often.

Q Are drugs of any help to an autistic child?

A Teachers and doctors agree that drugs are only of very limited use. Specialist teaching and training is of far more value in helping an autistic child to improve in relating to the outside world.

Q My seven-year-old autistic son attends a special school and is showing signs of improvement. Will he ever be able to live and work normally as an adult?

A A few autistic people do improve to this extent, but they remain inevitably a source of concern. Their difficulties do not arise from the work itself, which they can usually handle with ease, but from the social situations which arise before and after work, which distress and confuse them. But autistic people can earn a living as builders' labourers, accountancy clerks and piano tuners—all occupations demanding attention to detail without adding the burden of heavy responsibility.

The word 'autism' is used to describe an extremely complex form of mental handicap. It is taken from the Greek word 'autos', meaning 'self', and means being turned in upon the self.

It has been a recognized—that is to say medically classified—condition for over 40 years. In 1943, an American psychiatrist, Leo Kanner, first coined the word to describe the symptoms of a group of children whose common abnormalities of behaviour distinguished them sharply from the general mass of mentally handicapped children in his care. He identified what he considered to be the five most important symptoms common to them all, and from then on the condition became known as Kanner's syndrome, or 'infantile autism'.

Some years later, a working party of psychiatrists added four more symptoms to those selected by Kanner to make the 'nine points of autism' which for many years were used by doctors trying to diagnose the condition.

Attitudes to autism

Attitudes are different today. It is now believed that autism cannot be exactly separated into a category of its own. Many children possess autistic features who cannot be said to have Kanner's syndrome. Such children still need, however, the highly specialized education essential to the truly autistic, though 15 years ago they would have slipped through the diagnostic net.

Symptoms

What most parents usually notice first in their young autistic child is the inability to look others in the eye—an autistic child tends to look past the shoulder of whoever is speaking to them in a way which, if he or she were older, might well be thought impolite.

In fact, this puzzling aloofness is only the tip of the iceberg. As the toddler develops, the parents slowly realize that he or she is unable to participate in *any* normal social behaviour.

Tantrums

An autistic child's fits of screaming and trantrums far outdo in length and volume those of even the most violent normal toddler. This is at least partly because autistic children, while seeing and hearing normally, appear to be unable to make sense of what they see and hear. Their everyday world becomes terrifying.

Autistic children generally need special education with creative, supervised play. Support and understanding are required to prevent them withdrawing.

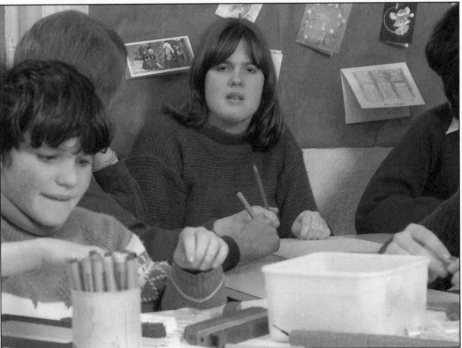

Brian Nash

Nor is there any refuge in the world of the imagination. The autistic toddler does not develop 'pretend play'—a brick remains a brick, and can never be transformed into a garage or a fort.

Effect on speech

Abnormalities of language vary from total muteness (inability to speak) to a literal, pedantic use of words. An autistic child, asked 'What do you do if you cut yourself?', answered, 'I bleed!' Echolalia—repeating the question instead of answering it—is frequent.

Strange responses

Autistic children also exhibit strange fears—usually of totally harmless objects such as a bush or a box, but do not register fear when there is real danger. This is probably connected to their inability to make sense of the impressions they receive.

Other aspects are less easy to explain. Such children tend to be over-sensitive to certain sounds—one used to run away screaming in distress from the sound of cold water gushing into the washing machine.

Then there is the fascination with bright lights, or with strange objects such as bits of broken plastic or elastic bands. And as if this were not enough, an autistic child may well show a disturbing indifference to heat and cold—being capable, for instance of stewing in a hot bath without showing any reaction. Strangest of all, perhaps, are the odd body movements—grimaces, arm- or hand-flapping, jumping or springing from one foot to the other—which no-one can satisfactorily explain.

This drawing by a six-year-old autistic child shows a developed sense of colour.

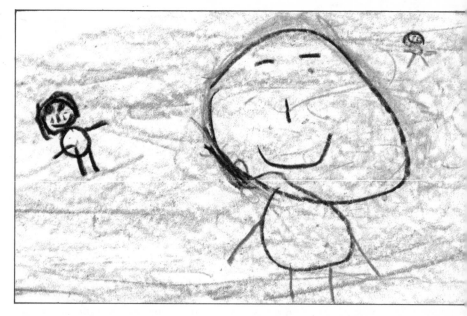

Types of autistic child

If all autistic children displayed all these symptoms, the condition would be much easier to diagnose. They do not, however, and the worried parent or relative can be even more confused by the fact that their child looks perfectly normal, even exceptionally beautiful and intelligent.

Just to throw everyone off the scent still further, many autistic children possess what are known as 'islands of normality'. These islands of normality usually affect activities where the development of language and certain other skills are not necessary—such as music, maths, or art. A child who is incapable of uttering a single spontaneous word may be a near – genius at mathematics, or have an extraordinary memory.

These islands of normality have even led parents of young autistic children to believe that they had an exceptionally

The drawings of this autistic six-year-old are more typical of a child of four.

gifted child, putting all other oddities of behaviour down to the quirks of genius until the increasing number of 'quirks' eventually disillusioned them.

Such children, who seem to stand astride the dividing line between normality and abnormality, if such a line exists, are sometimes able to live in ordinary society. But they remain immature, vulnerable, and in need of constant support.

A sheltered life

Other autistic children may develop a certain amount of useful speech, and acquire many practical skills, but cannot tolerate the whirl of everyday modern life.

Whilst they will always need to live in a sheltered environment, they are, however, capable of making important contributions to the success of that environment and of living full lives.

At the other end of the scale there are those who are so severely disturbed that their parents never had much doubt. At their worst, these children can turn a normal home to wreckage—tearing clothing, curtains, bedding, their own skin and hair.

Many have a minute sleep need, and remain hyperactive throughout the night, reducing parents to a pulp of shattered nerves. Still others—and these are perhaps the hardest to help—may be autistic in addition to other handicaps. Many partially deaf children, for instance, display autistic features.

Possible causes

We do not know the cause of autism. Over the years, many theories have been sug

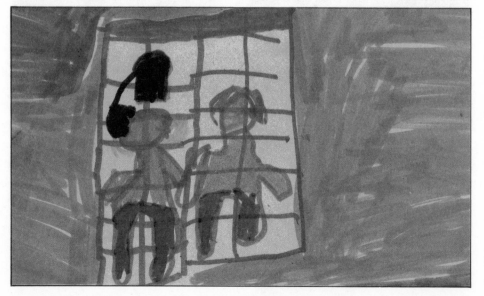

sted, but none proved conclusively.

Leo Kenner, having observed that the parents of his autistic children were all professional people, highly educated, but reticent in the interview situation, concluded that the children had withdrawn as a result of their parents' coldness.

This theory was in time ousted by others which at least had the merit of not adding to the parents' already considerable burden of guilt. In 1961, Bernard Rimland, another American psychiatrist, pointed out that three times as many boys as girls are born autistic; and that most autistic children are outstandingly beautiful and robust, with symmetrical features, dark complexions and long eyelashes.

In general, the evidence does bear him out, and the physical similarities between autistic children would seem to point to there being a physical cause for the condition—but there is still no actual proof.

Occasional improvement

Without knowing the cause it is, of course, impossible to find the cure. Most autistic children remain handicapped for life. Very rarely, a sudden easing of the symptoms' severity occurs, usually, oddly enough, when the child has been severely affected in the first instance.

It has been proved, too, that all autistic children do improve with special education, and parents should do everything to see that they receive it. No autistic child should be doomed to a mental sub-normality ward where, with no individual attention and affection, sedated and unmotivated, he or she can only get worse.

Teaching autistic children

Much of the pioneering work which established that these children need a specialized type of education was done in the UK and there are now schools in many countries. The improvement in the children who attended the early schools is well known and documented.

There cannot be one single teaching method or technique to be applied to all the children (like Braille for the blind, or sign language for the mute). Each child's highly individual needs and problems have to be assessed and treated. Different abilities have to be catered for in separate, individual learning programmes.

First steps

To start with, long-established techniques for behaviour management are employed to cope with the autistic abnormalities. The worst ones—tantrums, screaming fits, hyperactivity and obsessions—usually have to be dealt with first,

since of course they tend to stand in the way of real progress.

Language problems present the most fundamental obstacles to teaching, since they are linked with the problems of behaving properly and learning to think. They are, therefore, given constant attention. Advice and help are sought from audiology (hearing) clinics—and speech therapists, who test comprehension and expressive levels, and consider articulation problems.

Only after this is a language programme set up for the individual child. Language is concentrated on at all times—not just in the classroom. It is essential that all those engaged on teaching the child, at all levels, should themselves speak simply, using short sentences, and about things rather than ideas.

If autistic children remain mute beyond eight or nine years, there is little hope they can be taught any useful speech. Very rarely a child can be taught sign language, but this is exceptional.

Autistic children's lack of natural interest, motivation and concentration demand the teacher's careful organization of all daily situations in which the child finds itself. Normal children are taught to motivate themselves. Autistic children cannot—they have to be taught the *habit* of moving from one step to the next.

The degree of success depends of course upon the severity of the handicap. But some measure of it is possible for all the children.

Autistic children at home

It is very important that parents should be closely involved in the work and tech-

niques of the school. Autistic children are unable to transfer the training they have received in one environment to another, so that parents need to be familiar with the methods used in the school if the training is to be constant and unvaried. Otherwise, the child simply is not obtaining the maximum benefit from the special education.

There is tremendous joy to be found in teaching an autistic child at home. Autistic people can participate happily in many activities enjoyed by the normal—such as swimming, bowling, horse-riding and trampolining—and normal brothers and sisters can themselves benefit from helping out.

Again, it is important that parents should understand that no skill can be acquired in a rush—every activity has to be broken down into simple stages and infinite patience is necessary.

Outlook

Until as recently as 1974, the outlook for autistic children was bleak. One of the major problems was, and is, that they do not stop developing in their late teens, as do normal children, but can continue to improve, provided they are still being helped, well into their twenties.

School leaving age, however, is rigid, and although many schools or establishments teaching autistic children bent the rules and continued to care for the children for an extra year or so, in the end they had to leave still unable to cope.

Steps are beginning to be made—self-help communities, for instance—but more help is urgently needed.

Education should be continued beyond the teens for most autistics.

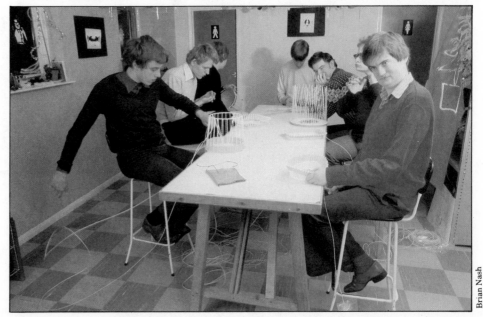

Brian Nash

Autonomic nervous system

Q Why is it that I often feel sleepy after I have had a big meal?

A Many of the processes of digestion depend on the autonomic nervous system. This has two sub-systems, the sympathetic, which is the system of action and activity, and the parasympathetic, which is generally concerned with relaxation. Digestion is mainly controlled by the parasympathetic system. So when it is at work the sympathetic system is less active than usual. This minor degree of parasympathetic overactivity and sympathetic underactivity combines to produce sleepiness.

Q Why does the hair 'stand on end' when people are frightened?

A Fright and other forms of stress influence the part of the nervous system known as the autonomic. This in turn controls the small muscles which do indeed lift the hair off the skin. At the same time, the pupils of the eyes will widen and sweating may start, particularly in the palms of the hands where the sweat glands are more directly controlled by the sympathetic nervous system than sweat glands in other parts of the body.

Q Are drugs which affect the autonomic nervous system dangerous?

A Like all drugs, those which affect the autonomic system must be carefully supervised. Nearly all of those in common use have a wide margin of safety. However, since the autonomic system controls functions basic to life (such as the heart and lungs), overdosage can be very serious.

Q Is it possible for the autonomic nervous system to be overactive?

A Some people do seem to have overactivity of the whole autonomic system, although at a low level. Such a patient may complain of such symptoms as palpitations and churning of the stomach. But it is a harmless condition and does not need treatment.

Breathing, digestion, heartbeat and many other vital bodily functions are managed for us, with no effort on our part, by the fascinating workings of the autonomic nervous system.

As we go about our lives, many processes within the body, such as breathing and digestion, keep us functioning smoothly. We usually take them for granted because they happen automatically. But all processes need some kind of controlling mechanism, and in the human body, two different systems provide this control.

'Automatic' control
One, the endocrine system, affects much of the body's chemistry through the production of hormones, which regulate growth and reproduction, among other functions. But, on the whole, hormone-controlled systems do not have to work quickly, or as spontaneously, as those controlled by the second system, autonomic nervous system.

This system, which is part of the whole nervous system, is mainly concerned with keeping up the automatic functions without deliberate mental or other effort on our part, of organs such as the heart, lungs, stomach, intestine, bladder, sex organs and blood vessels.

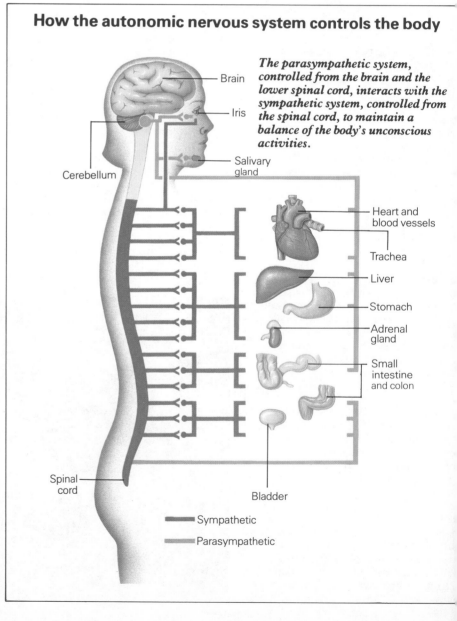

How the autonomic nervous system controls the body

The parasympathetic system, controlled from the brain and the lower spinal cord, interacts with the sympathetic system, controlled from the spinal cord, to maintain a balance of the body's unconscious activities.

Brain
Iris
Cerebellum
Salivary gland
Spinal cord
Heart and blood vessels
Trachea
Liver
Stomach
Adrenal gland
Small intestine and colon
Bladder

▬ Sympathetic
▬ Parasympathetic

ow it works

1 understanding of how the autonomic rvous system operates is vital to edicine mainly because its workings, rt chemical, part electrical, can be ntrolled or blocked by giving drugs. 1d this means, of course, that the organs influences can be controlled too.

Think of the nervous system as the ntrol system of the body. Thought and her conscious or 'deliberate' activities on in the brain hemispheres called the ghest' part of the system. The ones alt with here go on in the 'lower' parts the brain and in the spinal cord.

The actual process by which the ner-us system works is truly complicated, t in simple terms it can be thought of as ectrical signals being transmitted down rve fibres, each of which both end in 1d have nerve cells along their way.

The complexity and quantity of these lls and fibres within the body is astoni-ing: there are more than ten thousand illion in every one of us.

ells and axons

erve cells are the tiny bodies which her transmit or receive messages or nsations. The fibres, known in medical ience as axons, are the 'wires' along 1ich the impulses, or stimuli, travel to 1d from the control centres of the brain 1d spinal cord.

Nerve cells are not physically nnected to each other. There is a gap tween the ending of an axon and the ll itself called a synapse, across which e 'message' is carried by means of a emical. And this gap, with its chemical idge, is what enables doctors to control e system. For the action of these emical transmitters can be imitated th similar, man-made chemicals.

wo types of control

1e autonomic nervous system is divided :o two parts, known as the mpathetic and parasympathetic. Each es a different transmitter where the rve fibre reaches its target organ, each built differently, and each has a ferent effect on the organ it serves. Parasympathetic nerves serving, for ample, the bronchial airways leading and from the lungs, make them 1strict, or grow narrow. The mpathetic nerves leading to the same ea cause widening, that is dilating of e bronchial passages.

The chemical transmitter for parasym-thetic nerves is called acetylcholine, d the one for sympathetic nerves is led noradrenalin—close relative of renalin, the main hormone released to t the body's processes moving fast in ght or flight' situations.

Treatment of the autonomic system

Disease	Treatment
Common cold	Blocking drugs may 'dry up' a running nose or other mucus secretions. They act on the parasympathetic nerves
Asthma	Stimulant drugs are the mainstay of treatment. They act on the sympathetic nerves of the autonomic system
Ulcers (Stomach and duodenal)	The vagus nerve may be divided to reduce acid secretion
Angina	Sympathetic 'blocking' drugs are the non-surgical treatment
Heart attack	Sometimes a very slow heart rate may be improved with atropine—a parasympathetic 'blocking' drug
Abnormal heart rhythms (Palpitations)	Some abnormalities of the heart rhythms are treated with drugs which block the sympathetic system
Glaucoma (High pressure within the eye)	Parasympathetic stimulating drugs constrict the pupil of the eye, which helps lower the pressure
Hypertension	Sympathetic blocking drugs are one major form of therapy.

Manipulating the system

Armed with this knowledge, doctors have, for example, learnt how to success-fully treat asthma.

This is a drastic narrowing of the bronchial airways caused in the first place by allergic reaction to substances such as house dust. If the patient inhales a drug similar to noradrenalin, the sym-pathetic nerve system is assisted, the bronchial airways dilate, and the attack stops.

And when a chesty person is producing too much mucus, a drug which blocks the parasympathetic system may help the patient too.

Belladonna

A drug commonly used to block the para-sympathetic system is atropine. This used to be known as belladonna because beautiful ladies (in Italian *bella* means beautiful and *donna* means lady) put drops of atropine in their eyes to widen the pupils to increase their allure. The drug was extracted from, among other plants, deadly nightshade, which is also sometimes called belladonna.

However, if a patient is suffering from angina (poor delivery of oxygen to the heart), then a drug to block the sympathetic nervous system and noradrenalin activity may be used. It is not surprising that this sort of drug, called a beta blocker, sometimes causes asthma at the same time as relieving angina.

Surgery may even be used on the auto-nomic nervous system. The most usual such operation is a vagotomy, or cutting

of the vagus nerve, which is a large bundle of parasympathetic nerves in the chest. This reduces acid secretions in the stomach which in turn relieves gastric or duodenal ulcers.

Diseases of the autonomic system

The autonomic system itself rarely gives serious trouble, but one minor problem is relatively common—fainting.

Fainting attacks are technically called vaso-vagal attacks and the name gives a clue to the mechanism. 'Vasa' are blood vessels and the vagus is the major nerve of the parasympathetic system. Relative over-activity of the parasympathetic system causes dilation, or widening of the blood vessels, particularly the smallest arteries (the arterioles). As a result, the blood pressure falls and there is a reduction in the flow of blood to the brain, causing loss of consciousness.

The treatment is simple. Once the patient is laid flat, a position to which he or she is quite likely to have fallen in any case, then blood no longers pools in the lower part of the body, so that blood flow and consciousness returns to the brain.

More serious problems

Occasionally, the autonomic nervous system may cease to work either wholly or in part. A disease of the autonomic nerves may occur on its own, and it is not simple to treat. However, the most common cause of serious problems is diabetes (the production of dangerously high sugar levels in the body) and this condition can normally be effectively controlled by modern drug therapy.

B-vitamins

Q I'm on the Pill and suffering from headaches and depression. Would I benefit from a general vitamin supplement or would I be better taking one of the B vitamins?

A As the Pill often results in pyridoxine deficiency, you can offset this by taking more of this vitamin, and adding brown rice, liver, chicken, mackerel, peanuts, brewer's yeast and wheat germ to your diet. Start with 2-5 mg, and increase the daily allowance if symptoms do not disappear. For a general supplement, take B complex capsules.

Q Will heavy drinking cause a vitamin B deficiency?

A Yes! Heavy drinking impairs the body's ability to use thiamine, one of the B vitamins. The poor concentration, fatigue and weight loss alcoholics suffer from may be due as much to thiamine deficiency as excess drinking. Drink less, or if you find it difficult to cut down, make sure your diet contains more milk, wholemeal bread, beef, fortified cornflakes and peanuts. Brewer's yeast will provide thiamine in concentrated form.

Q My children will only eat white rice and white bread. Could they get beriberi?

A It's extremely unlikely. The association of beriberi with white cereals is not due to eating the cereals, it is due to eating virtually nothing else. White rice and bread provide carbohydrate intake not a source of thiamine. Wheat flour (and hence bread) is by law supplemented with thiamine, and most diets contain many other sources of thiamine, which makes this dietary deficiency very rare.

Q I have been prescribed a vitamin B supplement. Is it possible to take too much?

A Theoretically no, since the vitamin is not stored in the body and any excess is excreted. But *very* large doses might constitute a major challenge to your system, and it is possible that some sort of toxic effect could follow.

Vitamin B is essential for the regulation of the body's processes. Unlike most other vitamins, it is not stored in t. body and needs to be consumed daily. Fortunately, it is present in a wide variety of foods.

Vitamin B is a complex of at least eight separate water-soluble vitamins: B1 (thiamin), B2 (riboflavin), B3 (niacin), folic acid (folacin), B6 (pyridoxine), B12 (cyanocobalamin), biotin and pantothenic acid. They can be obtained in adequate supplies by eating a good balanced diet, since B vitamins are present in a wide variety of foods.

However, B vitamins can be easily destroyed, and their absorption and use by the body is affected by drugs or excessive alcohol; if a deficiency occurs, disease can result.

Uses
The B vitamins have a number of uses in the body. They act with enzymes to maintain chemical actions, particularly to do with breaking down food. They are involved in the process of providing the body with energy, basically by converting carbohydrates into glucose. And they are vital in the digestion and use of fats and protein.

The B vitamins are also necessary for the normal functioning of the nervous system, and for the maintenance of muscle tone in the gastrointestinal tract.

Pyridoxine (B6) assists in hormone production, and it must be present for the production of antibodies and red blood cells. Folic acid and B12 are also involved with red cell formation. Riboflavin maintains the skin, liver and eyes. Other vitamins in this group also perform functions necessary to good health.

Sources
Almost all the B vitamins occur in brewer's yeast (the richest natural source), liver and other organ meats, and wholegrain cereals. Cow's milk, eggs, nuts, legumes and green leafy vegetables are also rich in many of the B vitamins.

B vitamins, particularly biotin, are also produced by bacteria in the human intestine. These bacteria grow best on milk, sugar and small amounts of fat in the diet.

How vitamin B is lost
The body does not store vitamin B, making regular daily replenishment vital. Because the B vitamins dissolve in water, much of their nutritive value can be lost in cooking. Premature harvesting, long and improper storage also cause vitamin B loss. Thiamin is most affected,

and nicotinic acid the least.

Food processing also affects the B vi mins in foods. Milling wheat to produ white flour results in a lowering of t thiamin and nicotinic acid conte Milling and the extraction of bran a germ from rice means that polished r contains less thiamin. Cereals which ha been processed have fewer vitamins.

Canned meats contain fewer vitami than home-cooked meats. Light affe riboflavin in bottled milk.

Ideally, all vegetables and fru should be ripened on the plant and eat raw and with the skin still immediately after being harvested. Sir such ideal circumstances are impracti for most people, attempts should be ma to buy fresh produce only in quantit which can be used promptly, and to co them (preferably by steaming, not bo ing in water) as little as possible. Ofte frozen vegetables and fruits contain mo vitamin B than those improperly shipp and stored.

Deficiency
Deficiency of vitamin B can occur bo from low intakes and from its destru tion, for example, by excessive alcohol sugar intake.

A lack of vitamin B can lead to vario conditions, including beriberi. This rarely found in developed countries.

Wet beriberi arises from a thiamin-fr diet, and is characterized by eden waterlogging and swelling of the boc Dry beriberi occurs through a thiam deficiency but the deterioration in heal is slower and edema may not appea Both forms of beriberi affect the functio ing of the nervous system, but the bra is usually unimpaired.

Infantile beriberi is a disease whi affects children breast-fed by thiami deficient mothers; here, brain malfur tion exists, together with convulsior uneasiness and loss of voice. In ra cases, beriberi might arise followir fever, pregnancy or hard physical work

In the United States, thiamin de ciency occurs almost exclusively alcoholics, primarily due to a poor dieta intake. However, it has also been demo strated that severe alcoholism affec intestinal absorption of thiamin.

Pellegra is another vitamin B-relate condition present in areas where there poverty and famine, but it also occurs

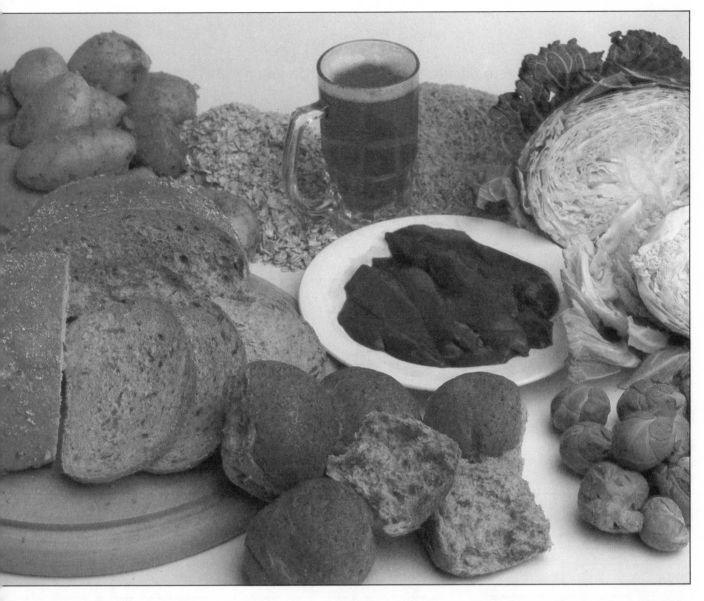

A varied diet is the best guarantee of adequate vitamin B—which is present in many foods. Even beer is a source of nicotinic acid.

...eople whose diets consist mainly of fats ...nd carbohydrates, or alcohol. It is a ...esult of inadequate supply of nicotinic ...cid, and symptoms include burning and ...ching, skin blotches, weakness, diarrhea ...nd depression.

Pernicious anemia is a disease which ...ccurs mainly in people who lack the ...bility to absorb and utilize vitamin B12, ...nd vegans, who shun milk, eggs, meat ...nd fish completely. B12 can be taken in ...ill form or by injection, and eating raw ...ver is also a cure.

Sores on the skin, often at the corner of ...he mouth, are usually caused by a defi- ...ency in riboflavin. Inadequate ribofla- ...in also causes lesions of the cornea.

A deficiency of folacin is indicated by a ...ery red tongue, diarrhea and sometimes anemia, poor growth and greying hair.

Pyridoxine (vitamin B6) deficiency can cause anemia, and irritability, kidney stones, and muscle twitching.

Lack of biotin can lead to tiredness, depression, nausea, skin problems, and aches and pains.

A deficiency of pantothenic acid is rare, because it is found in most foods.

When a supplement is necessary

The need for B vitamins increases during infection or stress, as well as during pregnancy and in the presence of certain drugs.

The contraceptive pill creates a greater need for pyridoxine. Women on the Pill who experience headaches or depression may need to add it to their diet.

Pregnant women can benefit from taking two B vitamins. If there are early signs of toxemia, such as swelling feet, ankles and fingers, an increased dose of pyridoxine can be taken, and should be continued during breast-feeding. It is also used as an anti-sickness treatment.

Pregnant women should also take folic acid, which is often given in a combined pill with iron supplements. Folic acid deficiency is the most common vitamin deficiency in the US, but is easily corrected with supplements.

Folic acid is involved in the making of red blood cells: the body has to produce more of these cells in pregnancy to help with the nourishment and development of the fetus. Without folic acid, a pregnant woman will risk such complications as toxemia, premature birth and hemorrhaging, all the result of a condition called megaloblastic anemia, which causes tiredness and weakness.

Breast-feeding mothers are advised to increase their niacin intake.

Doctors recommend additional pyridoxine to alleviate the symptoms of pre-

Vitamin B

How much vitamin B complex do you need in a day?

Age group	Thiamin (mg)	Riboflavin (mg)	Nicotinic acid (mg)
Babies under 1 year	0.3 to 0.5	0.4 to 0.6	5 to 8
Children aged 1 to 6	0.7 to 0.9	0.8 to 1.1	9 to 12
Children aged 7 to 10	1.2	1.2	16
Male teenagers	1.4 to 1.5	1.5 to 1.8	18 to 20
Female teenagers	1.1 to 1.2	1.3 to 1.4	14 to 16
Men	1.4	1.6	18
Women	1.0	1.2	13
Pregnant women	1.3	1.5	15
Lactating women	1.3	1.7	17

Vitamin B in the diet

You only need to eat a normal, balanced diet in order to satisfy your daily requirement of Vitamin B. As you can see from the chart below, a variety of foods contain vitamin B components. Vitamin amounts are given in mg. Quantities of pyridoxine, B12, folic acid, pantothenic acid and biotin required are miniscule and are present in an everyday diet.

Thiamin

1 large slice of wholewheat bread	0.15
114 g (4 oz) cured, cooked ham	0.6
114 g (4 oz) wheatflakes cereal	0.6
70 g (½ cup) blackberries	0.2

Riboflavin

114 g (4 oz) Brussels sprouts or cabbage	1.0
1 wholewheat bread roll	0.1
114 g (4 oz) liver	3.5
1 egg	0.25

Nicotinic acid

a small glass of milk	1.8
114 g (4 oz) cheddar cheese	7.0
114 g (4 oz) beef	8.0
½ cup roasted salted peanuts	1.2

Sources of vitamin B

	Milk	Tea/coffee	Wholewheat bread	Cheese	Liver	Potatoes	Eggs	Peanuts	Wholegrain cereals	Chicken	Green vegetables	Kidney	Beef	Brewer's yeast	Beer
Thiamin (B1)	X		X			X		X	X		X		X	X	
Riboflavin (B2)	X			X	X	X	X		X	X	X	X			
Nicotinic acid (B3)	X	X		X		X	X	X	X		X		X		X
Folic acid			X		X				X		X	X		X	
Pyridoxine (B6)			X		X	X			X			X	X	X	
B12	X				X							X	X	X	
Biotin	X				X		X	X				X		X	
Pantothenic acid	X		X		X		X	X	X	X	X	X	X	X	

menstrual syndrome: headaches, depression and painful breasts.

Finally, the use of cortisone drugs or other steroids, and the hormone estrogen, and dieting, create a need for pyridoxine; it can also be helpful for acne and other skin conditions, and to alleviate the side-effects of the menopause.

Toxicity

Overconsumption is rare with B vitamins, since they are not stored in the body. However, excessive amounts of nicotinic acid (a form of niacin) may cause flushing, headache, cramps and nausea. Too much folacin may mask the presence of pernicious anemia. Large supplements of vitamin B6 have been shown to cause sensory nerve damage, resulting in a crippling loss of mobility.

Other B vitamins

There are several other substances which are considered by some to be B vitamins. B13 (orotic acid) has been synthesized in Europe and is found in organically grown root vegetables. B15 (pangamic acid) has been tested in the USSR, but little is known about it in the US. B17 (laetrile) is the one B vitamin which does not occur naturally in brewer's yeast. Choline and inositol are closely associated with biotin. PABA (para-aminobenzoic acid) stimulates the intestinal bacteria to produce other B vitamns, folic acid and pantothenic acid.

Some of these substances have been promoted by faddists as cures for various ailments. Scientific evidence is lacking, however, and a physician's advice should be sought before taking very large doses of vitamin B—or other vitamins.